"In this wonderful, easy-to-read-and-use book, Carol Krucoff has gracefully and intelligently integrated several important healing traditions in order to bring relief to those suffering from neck and shoulder pain and the pain of stress. I recommend it enthusiastically as a friendly vehicle anyone can use to explore and experience the amazing power and healing potential of these human bodies."

> —Jeffrey Brantley, MD, director of the Mindfulness-Based Stress Reduction Program at Duke Integrative Medicine, and coauthor of *Five Good Minutes® in Your Body*

"Unlike modern medicine, which often does little more than suppress the symptoms of neck problems with painkillers, yoga can get at the root causes of pain. In this wonderful book, Krucoff demonstrates safe, gentle, and effective strategies to lessen neck and shoulder discomfort. Be careful, though—yoga's side effects include peace of mind, improved mood, and better sleep. You could get hooked!"

> —Timothy McCall, MD, medical editor of *Yoga Journal* and author of *Yoga as Medicine*

"What a gift Krucoff has given us! These practices guide us in both postural and emotional healing of the neck and shoulders by allowing the energy to flow freely, uniting head to body and head to heart. This brings about a sense of balance and ease, reminding us of our joyful nature."

> —Nischala Joy Devi, author *The Healing Path of Yoga* and *The Secret Power of Yoga*

healing yoga
for neck &
shoulder pain

Easy, Effective Practices for
Releasing Tension & Relieving Pain

CAROL KRUCOFF, E-RYT

New Harbinger Publications, Inc.

Publisher's Note

This publication is designed to provide accurate and authoritative information in regard to the subject matter covered. It is sold with the understanding that the publisher is not engaged in rendering psychological, financial, legal, or other professional services. If expert assistance or counseling is needed, the services of a competent professional should be sought.

Distributed in Canada by Raincoast Books

Copyright © 2010 by Carol Krucoff
New Harbinger Publications, Inc.
5674 Shattuck Avenue
Oakland, CA 94609
www.newharbinger.com

Cover design by Amy Shoup
Text design by Michele Waters-Kermes
Acquired by Jess O'Brien
Edited by Nelda Street

FSC

Mixed Sources
Product group from well-managed
forests and other controlled sources

Cert no. SW-COC-002283
www.fsc.org
© 1996 Forest Stewardship Council

Library of Congress Cataloging-in-Publication Data

Krucoff, Carol.
    Healing yoga for neck and shoulder pain : easy, effective practices for releasing tension and relieving pain / Carol Krucoff ; foreword by Tracy W. Gaudet.
        p. cm.
    Includes bibliographical references.
    ISBN 978-1-57224-712-3
    1. Yoga--Therapeutic use. 2. Mind and body. I. Title.
    RM727.Y64K78 2010
    613.7'046--dc22
                        2010002488

12   11   10

10   9   8   7   6   5   4   3   2   1

First printing

In loving memory of Esther Myers,
gifted teacher, wise friend, and indomitable spirit

contents

Foreword   ix

Acknowledgments   xv

Introduction: Healing "Pain in the Neck"—and
Shoulders, Upper Back, Jaw, & Head, Too   1

chapter 1   The Science of Neck Pain & How Yoga Can Help   5

chapter 2   The Inside Story: Anatomy, Posture, & Pain   25

chapter 3   The Emotional Connection: The Role of Stress
& the Energetic Body in Neck & Shoulder Pain   41

chapter 4   Putting Your Head On Straight: Posture
Guidelines for Daily Life   57

chapter 5   Healing Yoga Practice to Prevent & Relieve
Neck & Shoulder Pain   71

1.   Centering   83

2.   Breath Awareness   84

3.   Body Scan   85

4.   Exhaling Tension   85

5.   Deep Abdominal Breath   86

6.   Neck Release   88

7.   Neck Stretch   89

8.   Upper Back and Shoulder Stretch   90

9.   Single-Knee-to-Chest Pose with
Ankle Circles   92

10.   Leg Stretch   93

11.   Both-Knees-to-Chest Pose   94

12.   Cat Pose and Dog Tilt   96

13.   Spinal Balance   98

14.   Child's Pose   100

15.   Mountain Pose   102

16.   Standing Salutation   104

17.   Mountain Pose Variation—
Arm Up/Head Turn   106

18.   Tree Pose   108

19.   Puppy Dog   110

20.   Gentle Twist   111

21.   Seated Mountain Pose   112

22.   Shoulder Shrugs   114

23.	Shoulder Clock	116
24.	Hug Arms	118
25.	Angel Wings	120
26.	Angel-Wing Circles	121
27.	Seated Back Bend	122
28.	Head Turn	123
29.	Ear to Shoulder	124
30.	Bobblehead	126
31.	Wrist, Arm, and Side Stretch	126
32.	Cow's-Face Arms	128
33.	Lion's Face	129
34.	Crocodile Pose	130
35.	Modified Locust Pose	131
36.	Baby Cobra	132
37.	Bridge Pose	134
38.	Savasana	136
chapter 6	Neck Check: Eight Essential Self-Care Strategies for Lasting Relief	141
	Resources	151
	References	157

foreword

Our bodies are always speaking to us—but at first in whispers. If we don't listen and respond to these whispers, eventually our bodies will begin to scream. This is a truth I've seen over and over again in my work as a physician specializing in integrative medicine, a new approach to medical care that focuses on the whole person, recognizing that the subtle interactions of mind, body, spirit, and community have a direct impact on our vitality and well-being.

And I've seen this not just in my patients but also in my own life—specifically as it related to a severe case of neck pain I experienced in the mid-1990s, when I had the amazing opportunity to be named the founding executive director for the Program in Integrative Medicine at the University of Arizona. Dr. Andrew

Weil was the program's visionary, and it was my job to turn this vision into a reality. We had just nine months from the time I moved to Tucson until the first class of physicians arrived. There was no curriculum, no faculty, no clinic—indeed no process for recruiting or selecting the physicians! Somewhere in the course of those nine months, I began experiencing something that had never happened to me before. One day I would be fine as I went about my life, and then the next morning, I would wake up with excruciating neck pain. My neck (usually one side more than the other) was in such an extreme spasm that I literally couldn't turn my head. And I felt as if this pain truly came from nowhere. I never felt it coming on, and I was completely unaware of anything in my life or lifestyle that was contributing to or triggering these disturbing spasms. As you can imagine, this neck pain was quite disruptive, since it made anything that required turning my head a problem and since it was so *painful*, inhibiting such essential activities as driving a car and having a normal, socially appropriate conversation.

When I reflect back on this now, I have to laugh at how oblivious I was to the mind-body connection underlying my neck pain. If I had actually been paying attention to my *body*, I would have begun to notice (and subsequently did) changes in my neck that were, at first, subtle about a week before my symptoms peaked. And if I had been paying attention to my *mind*, I could have predicted the likelihood that my neck would take this path about a week prior to the first sign from my body. If I had known what to do, I could have intervened at either of those times and, most likely, averted this debilitating neck pain with very simple, yet incredibly powerful, yoga-based techniques. And last, had I been proactive about my self-care and taken small steps every day to optimize my health, particularly for my neck and shoulders, I would rarely have needed to do anything more.

Healing Yoga for Neck and Shoulder Pain teaches exactly what I wish I had known back in those days at the University of Arizona, what I'm so fortunate to know now. In this comprehensive book, Carol Krucoff draws on her many years of experience and teaching to show you how you can use yoga not only to help alleviate and eliminate significant pain, but also to return you to levels of health and vitality you may have forgotten were possible. I'm honored to have Carol as both a friend and colleague, and in her work as a yoga therapist with Duke Integrative Medicine, I have personally seen her remarkable outcomes with patients too numerous to count. Carol not only is skilled in this work with patients but also knows exactly how to teach others how to use the tools of yoga to heal themselves. Her approach has transformed the lives of people struggling with neck and shoulder pain. And now her book teaches you what you need to know to do this for yourself.

The benefits of Carol's approach to yoga are manyfold. First, this approach is fabulous at helping you reconnect with your body. You can begin to become much more aware of the state of your body, and respond to the early signs and symptoms rather than wait until they're so severe they can no longer be ignored, as I used to do. Yoga, and particularly Carol's approach to working with this ancient healing tradition, allows you to hone your skills of reconnecting to your body and listening to its whispers so you can respond to its needs before any problems escalate.

These practices also give you the opportunity to tune in to the whispers of your soul, or your nonphysical self. In my life, and in the lives of many people, high levels of stress and tension most often precede neck and shoulder pain. By learning to become more aware of your mental and psychological states, you have the opportunity to intervene proactively and avert a bigger, more full-blown pain syndrome down the road.

Grounded in this greater awareness, the practical approaches based in ancient yoga traditions are the most powerful part of what Carol teaches. Let's face it: if, after reading this book, you've become more aware of the physical and mental precursors to your pain but can't do anything to avert it, we haven't done you much of a service! And, on those occasions when we are in acute pain, these effective self-care strategies are absolutely invaluable.

You will begin to notice the effect of these approaches in two main ways. Over time, as you practice the yoga poses and breathing, you will notice the impact of greater strength and increased flexibility, as well as much improved posture and overall alignment of your physical body. You will also be very aware of the impact on your mental processes, particularly the deep sense of relaxation and stress reduction the yoga practice cultivates, as well as the opportunity to simply reconnect with yourself. In our busy, overcommitted 24/7 culture, this is a precious and essential self-care strategy.

What's often surprising to people who work with Carol's approach is the degree to which their bodies and minds are also affected in the everyday moments of their lives. Integrating yoga into your life in what I refer to as the "informal practice" has a more subtle but equally significant impact on your life and health. These strategies work synergistically to provide effective and often dramatic relief of neck and shoulder pain, as well as greater levels of energy and peace of mind.

Healing Yoga for Neck and Shoulder Pain gives you the self-care tools necessary to become more aware of your body and your soul, and teaches you very effective strategies to support each of them in building strength and flexibility, and reducing tension and stress. The end result? Relief and, we hope, elimination of your pain, plus increased energy and vitality—all as a result of simple practices that you yourself can do and can sustain across your lifetime. Now that's taking care of your health at its finest!

—Tracy Gaudet, MD
   Executive Director, Duke Integrative Medicine
   Assistant Professor of Obstetrics and Gynecology, Duke
      University School of Medicine
   Durham, North Carolina

acknowledgments

I am grateful for the wisdom, kindness, and support of many wonderful people who have contributed to this book. In particular, I would like to thank highly accomplished and accredited physical therapist and yoga therapist, Matthew J. Taylor, PT, Ph.D., for taking time from his busy rehabilitation practice and work as president of the International Association of Yoga Therapists to review this manuscript and offer excellent feedback. Thanks to my Yoga for Seniors partner and spiritual sister Kimberly Carson, MPH, E-RYT, for helping shape some of the meditations offered in these chapters, and thanks also to my teacher and dear friend Nischala Joy Devi for sharing her deep insights into the yogic perspective on healing. Thanks to artist Sarah Craige for her skillful photography on which the posture illustrations are based.

My extraordinary colleagues at Duke Integrative Medicine are a living example of how medical care can do more than just treat disease, how it can truly optimize health. Working with this incredibly talented group of healers is an ongoing inspiration, and I am honored that our executive director, the incomparable and visionary Tracy Gaudet, MD, has graced this book with a foreword. I treasure her friendship and support.

Thanks to the outstanding editorial team at New Harbinger, particularly Wendy Millstine for initiating the conversation that resulted in this book, Jess O'Brien and Jess Beebe for their insightful advice, and Nelda Street for her meticulous copyediting. Thanks, too, to Lynn Shwadchuck for her lovely illustrations, which help bring the postures to life.

I am grateful to the many yoga teachers I've studied with over more than thirty years—in particular my mentor Esther Myers and her teacher Vanda Scaravelli. I've also been greatly influenced by the teaching of T. K. V. Desikachar, Larry Payne, Gary Kraftsow, Leslie Kaminoff, Todd Norian, Richard Freeman, Erich Schiffmann, Kathy Hallen, Molly Drake, Angela Farmer, and Victor van Kooten. I continually learn from my yoga students and yoga therapy clients, and offer them sincere thanks for allowing me the gift of service. Special thanks to the staff and members of the Gerofit gerontology rehabilitation program at the Durham Veterans Administration Medical Center, who gave me the opportunity to be "the yoga lady" and realize the profound transformational power yoga can have for *every* body—regardless of health status or physical ability.

Immeasurable thanks to my friends and family for their love and support, and a warm belly rub to our beagle Sheba—exemplar of healthy habits like frequent stretching, napping, and tail wagging. For the blessings of my remarkable husband Mitchell, son Max, and daughter Rae, I am profoundly, humbly, and eternally grateful.

introduction: healing "pain in the neck"— and shoulders, upper back, jaw, & head, too

If your neck is chronically tense and tight, and if the muscles in your upper back and shoulders often feel as hard as a rock, you're not alone. In our high-stress, hurried, 24/7 world—filled with work deadlines, financial pressures, "terror alerts," and sleeplessness—many of us feel the weight of the world on our shoulders. Add to this emotional tension the postural stress of spending most of our days sitting, typically doing activities that round our bodies forward—such as computer work, driving, and reading—and all too often, the result is a serious pain in the neck.

And the problem doesn't stop here. Many people don't realize that chronic neck pain is associated with a constellation of related disorders, including headache; jaw discomfort; and upper back, shoulder, and arm soreness. That tingling in your fingers, ache in your arms, and vice-like sensation of pressure encircling your skull may all be related to neck pain. In addition, the slumped posture that can lead to neck pain may compress internal organs, contributing to respiratory, circulatory, and digestive problems as well.

Yet modern medicine offers most people struggling with neck pain and its associated disorders little other than painkilling medications that address the *symptoms*, but not the *cause*, of their problems. In fact, a popular treatment, the cervical collar, is unlikely to help in relieving neck pain, according to a report published in *Spine* journal (Hurwitz et al. 2008). Other common remedies that are also unlikely to help include ultrasound, electrical muscle stimulation, and most injection therapies (ibid.).

Experts are now recognizing that, for most people suffering from neck pain and its associated disorders, the most helpful strategy is self-care. Yoga is a powerful form of self-care on several levels:

Physical: Yoga poses help stretch tight muscles and strengthen weak ones, cultivating flexibility, stability, and ease of movement. Yoga also teaches proper alignment, which helps you learn how to sit and stand with good posture, easing strain on your neck and shoulders.

Psychological: Yoga is a potent stress reliever that teaches you how to relax and connect to an inner sense of peace. In addition, the process of self-discovery that begins on the yoga mat helps you understand yourself better, shedding light on your habitual stress patterns and emotional reactions—which typically translates into learning healthier ways of relating to the world in everyday life.

Energetic: Yoga breathing helps enhance vital energy and recharges your entire system. Yoga postures can help release physical and emotional energy blockages, facilitating a healthy flow of *prana* (vital energy) throughout every cell. The yogic approach of balancing effort with relaxation can help you learn how to avoid expending energy in unnecessary ways so that you stop spinning your wheels and use only what you need.

This book is designed to empower you with safe, effective self-care strategies gleaned from the ancient practice of yoga and adapted to help heal our modern epidemic of neck and shoulder pain. It's based on my work with countless yoga students and yoga therapy clients, as well as my own struggles with neck pain. As a journalist who worked under deadline pressure at the *Washington Post* for ten years (from 1977 to 1987), I often experienced neck pain, which, at its worst, resulted in frequent headaches. This problem led me to yoga, whose therapeutic powers were so profound that I furthered my study of this holistic discipline to both heal myself and help teach others how to access yoga's extraordinary health benefits. Over time, I have virtually eliminated my own neck pain, and feel grateful to be able to share the myriad gifts of yoga with you.

the science of neck pain & how yoga can help

Whenever I teach a yoga class, I typically begin by asking students if they have any requests, if there are particular places in their bodies where they feel tension, tightness, or discomfort they'd like our session to address. The single most common reply is "neck and shoulders," which is the central reason for this book! Particularly in an evening class, where many students have come straight from work, tight shoulders, upper-back tension, and general neck pain are widespread.

In some people, stiffness in these areas is so pronounced that it becomes disabling. A prime example is a student I'll call Susan, whose neck and shoulder tension was so severe that she had trouble turning her head to change lanes when driving. This made getting behind the wheel increasingly frightening. An office manager in her mid-forties, Susan sat hunched over a computer most of the day. Her posture was poor, with her chin jutted forward and her upper back rounded, and she carried so much tension in her upper body that her shoulders were raised up near her ears.

Fear brought Susan to yoga. After narrowly escaping a car accident, which she blamed on her inability to turn her head, she was so scared that she vowed to take action. A friend suggested that Susan accompany her to yoga class, and when Susan walked in the door, you could see the tension etched in her face. At first, when she lay on her back at the beginning of class, Susan's neck was so stiff that she could barely rock her head from side to side. Her shoulders were so tight that she couldn't raise her arms all the way up over her head. When I gently touched her shoulders and invited her to relax her muscles, there was very little movement; chronic tension had forged a kind of rigid "body armor" that resisted letting go.

Over time, with regular yoga practice, this rigidity began to soften. Like many people who habitually carry tension in their bodies, Susan was surprised to discover all the places in her body where she stored stress. And she was even more astonished that she could learn how to consciously relax and release these tense muscles, especially those in her neck, shoulders, jaw, and face. Her posture improved, and she found herself able to do things that were previously difficult or painful, such as reaching back to hook her bra and turning to look at something behind her. Now, after three years of regular yoga practice, Susan looks and feels wonderful, with beautiful posture that gives her an air of confidence, relaxed shoulders, smiling eyes, and a flexible neck that turns smoothly and easily. In the rare instances when she feels any twinge of neck or shoulder pain, Susan uses yoga postures and breathing practices to unlock tension and find relief.

These changes didn't happen overnight. Yoga takes time, patience, and practice. But this ancient, holistic self-care discipline offers profound tools for healing on many levels—providing remedies that are practical, effective, and lasting. And yoga's benefits can be particularly helpful in relieving a complex, multifaceted ailment such as neck and shoulder pain. In this chapter we'll explore what modern medical science has learned about neck pain and its associated disorders, including why it's such a common problem, who's at risk, and what treatments work best. I'll also offer an overview of the ancient Indian practice of yoga, examining why and how it can offer you profound healing from neck and shoulder pain.

the science of neck pain

While back pain generally commands more attention—in part, because it results in more work-related disability—neck pain is nearly as common. Consider these statistics from the Bone and Joint Decade 2000–2010 Task Force on Neck Pain and Its Associated Disorders (Haldeman, Carroll, and Cassidy 2008), an international group of clinician-scientists established in 2000 as part of the World Health Organization's global initiative focusing on musculoskeletal disorders:

+ Most people can expect to experience some degree of neck pain in their lifetimes (Haldeman et al. 2008).

+ Up to 70 percent of people report experiencing neck pain over the past year, and up to 45 percent report experiencing neck pain over the past month (Hogg-Johnson et al. 2008).

+ About 5 percent of North Americans report being disabled because of neck pain, and another 10 percent report experiencing low-level disability along with high-intensity neck pain (Lidgren 2008). In Europe, surveys show that chronic or persistent neck pain affects 10 to 20 percent of the population (ibid.).

+ Each year, 11 to 14.1 percent of workers report being limited in their activities because of neck pain (Côté et al. 2008). Neck pain is common in all occupational categories, and worker's compensation data appears to significantly underestimate the burden of neck pain in workers (ibid.).

+ Most people with neck pain do not experience a complete resolution of symptoms (Haldeman et al. 2008). Between 50 and 85 percent of those initially experiencing neck pain will report neck pain again one to five years later (ibid.).

Neck pain and its associated disorders—including headache and pain radiating into the upper back and arms—are much more common than anyone previously believed, according to the Task Force report, which was published in a special supplement to *Spine* journal (Lidgren 2008). Indeed, neck-related pain has become a major cause of disability around the world, according to these experts, who noted that the problem was not well understood and was, in many cases, very difficult to manage.

risk factors for neck pain

After undertaking a comprehensive review of the scientific literature on neck pain, as well as conducting several original research
projects, the Task Force concluded that neck pain has a "multifac-
torial etiology" (Hogg-Johnson et al. 2008); or in layman's terms, a
variety of risk factors can contribute to this problem. Some factors
that put you at risk for neck pain are outside of your control,
including the following (ibid.):

Age: The risk for neck pain increases with age up to a
peak in midlife (forty to fifty-four) and then declines in
later years.

Gender: The relationship between gender and neck pain
appears to vary depending on the kind of neck pain.
Studies suggest that men are more likely to seek care at a
hospital for a neck sprain or injury, often related to a trau-
matic event like getting hurt while playing sports or doing
physical labor. In contrast, women showed higher rates of
visits to a health care center for neck pain, which was less
likely to be related to a single specific, problematic event.

Genetics: Heredity appears to play a role in neck pain,
although the mechanisms of this relationship are not
understood.

Other factors that affect a person's risk of neck pain are con-
trollable, including the following:

- *Smoking and environmental exposure to tobacco* increases
  the risk of neck pain, since this can reduce the oxygen

content in tissues and contribute to musculoskeletal problems (ibid.).

- *Workplace stress*, including high quantitative job demands, low social support at work, sedentary work position, repetitive work, and precision work all increase the risk of neck pain (Côté et al. 2008).

- *Physical activity participation* protects against neck pain, since regular exercisers tend to be more fit and resilient, and also improves the prognosis for recovery from neck pain (Hogg-Johnson et al. 2008).

Surprisingly, the Task Force found no evidence that common degenerative changes in the cervical spine are a risk factor for neck pain (ibid.). The phrase, "common degenerative changes," refers to the gradual deterioration of the cartilage that cushions the joints, which occurs with age. This condition, known as *osteoarthritis*, often called "wear-and-tear arthritis," is the most common form of arthritis. These age-related arthritic changes are a natural fact of life, and by age fifty to sixty, most people have degenerative changes in the spine (Haldeman 2008). In most people, this is a benign process. However, when seen on X-ray or MRI, these inevitable changes are typically labeled *degenerative joint disease*, a frightening-sounding diagnosis for something that's generally a harmless part of growing older. When you call something a "disease," it's natural to go looking for a cure, and a whole body of literature exists based on the assumption that persistent and disabling neck pain is associated with degenerative changes in the cervical spine. But since the Task Force found no evidence to support this assumption, they proposed a new way of looking at and labeling neck pain.

new conceptual model of neck pain

Rather than view neck pain as a disease, which often sends people on a fruitless search for a magic cure, the Task Force proposed a shift in perspective that considers neck pain a phenomenon of life impacted by risk factors, many of which we can control. Based on their extensive research, this new conceptual model centers on empowering individuals to participate in their own care.

In other words, if you're like the vast majority of people with neck pain, there are steps you can take to help protect yourself and avoid letting neck pain interfere with your life. For example, the Task Force found that, in general, those things that keep you moving are good, including exercise and manual therapy, an umbrella term for hands-on physical treatments such as massage, myofascial release, and joint manipulation.

In contrast, typically those things that stop you from moving are bad, including collars and bed rest. Some other treatments appear beneficial, the Task Force noted (Haldeman et al. 2008), including educational videos, low-level laser therapy, and acupuncture. Interventions that focus on regaining function and returning to work as soon as possible were generally more effective than those without that focus.

Top self-care practices include avoiding smoking, keeping physically active, and maintaining positive thought processes. Research indicates that people with poor psychological health, who tend to worry and become angry or frustrated in response to neck pain, had a poorer prognosis, while those who were more optimistic and had a coping style that involved self-assurance were more likely to experience pain relief (Côté et al. 2008). Yoga can be particularly beneficial since it keeps you physically active, relieves stress, and enhances mood.

red-flag symptoms

While self-care is the best treatment for the vast majority of people who experience neck pain, certain "red-flag" symptoms may be signs of more serious conditions—such as cancer, fracture, or infection—and indicate the need for medical attention. It's advisable to consult a health professional if you're concerned about your neck pain, and it's essential to seek medical attention if you have red-flag symptoms such as:

- Numbness, tingling, or weakness in your arm or hand

- Pain caused by an injury, accident, or blow

- Swollen glands or a lump in your neck

- Difficulty swallowing or breathing

Check with your physician, too, if you have a condition that may make you more prone to serious neck injury, such as previous neck surgery, history of cancer, inflammatory arthritis, or bone loss due to osteoporosis or corticosteroid treatment.

how yoga can help

Yoga is a profound system of holistic healing that originated more than five thousand years ago in India. The word "yoga" comes from the ancient Sanskrit word *yuj*, which means to "yoke" or "unite," and the practice is designed to unify many things. At the most basic level, yoga helps unite body and mind. At a deeper level, yoga seeks to unite the individual with the universal.

When people in the West say "yoga," they're commonly referring to *hatha yoga*, one branch of this ancient discipline that focuses on physical postures, breathing exercises, and meditation. Hatha yoga teaches you how to relax and release tension, as well as strengthen weak muscles and stretch tight ones. It also helps balance and integrate mind, body, and spirit in order to enhance energy flow and stimulate the body's own natural healing processes.

A common misconception is that yoga is only for the fit and flexible, and requires you to twist yourself into a pretzel and stand on your head. One of the most frequent comments I hear when people learn that I teach yoga is, "Oh, I could never do yoga; I'm not flexible enough," to which I typically reply, "That's like thinking your house is too messy to hire a maid."

In fact, the only prerequisite for practicing yoga is being able to breathe! I've taught yoga to people with a wide range of health challenges, including cancer, heart disease, osteoporosis, arthritis, blindness, fibromyalgia, back pain, congestive heart failure, and leg amputation. While advanced postures like headstand are part of the yoga practice for some people, they're by no means required. Your yoga practice should be tailored to fit your own abilities and needs. For many people, yoga involves simple yet powerful meditative movements that anyone can do.

Yoga Is Medicine

When most people think of medicine, they visualize something material, like a pill to be popped, a liquid to be swallowed, or an injection to be endured. Some might also consider surgery, tests, or procedures to be medicine, since these high-tech maneuvers can help diagnose and treat disease. But the ancient yogis realized a truth that modern medicine now confirms: simple movement offers profound healing benefits. Today, this notion is embraced by traditional healers and modern scientists, Eastern and Western physicians alike: appropriate movement enhances health, while inactivity impairs it.

In other words, movement *is* medicine. And it's a medicine that's extremely effective, free (or at least inexpensive), low risk, abundantly available, socially acceptable, and simple to do. The main "side effect" is looking and feeling better. In fact, Dr. Robert Butler, founding director of the National Institute on Aging, is fond of saying, "If exercise could be packed in a pill, it would be the single most widely prescribed, and beneficial, medicine in the nation" (Butler 2009). All it takes to achieve substantial health benefits is regular practice.

Over the last few decades, Western medicine has increasingly recognized the healing power of movement and prescribed physical activity as a safe and effective treatment to help prevent, relieve, and sometimes even cure a host of disorders. Solid scientific evidence (U.S. Department of Health and Human Services 2008) documents exercise's therapeutic benefits in reducing the risk of, or helping heal, more than two dozen conditions, including heart disease, diabetes, certain cancers (colon, breast, pancreatic, and prostate), hypertension, arthritis, depression, osteoporosis, high cholesterol, stroke, asthma, sleep apnea, and even sexual dysfunction.

Appropriate movement enhances health, while inactivity impairs it.

Physical activity, in the form of postures and breathing practices, is a central component of yoga, but the practice is much more than just a workout. Yoga is a powerful form of mind-body medicine that approaches health in a holistic manner, recognizing that physical ailments also have emotional and spiritual components. For example, neck pain may involve a wide array of contributing factors ranging from poor posture, weak muscles, and repetitive behaviors to stress, anxiety, and fear. Yoga is based on an appreciation for the interconnectedness of all aspects of our being, and seeks to unify and integrate the wide variety of factors that affect our health. At its heart, the practice is a comprehensive system for self-development and transformation.

Yoga offers a variety of techniques for healing, including:

Postures: Yoga poses help stretch and strengthen your body and are grounded in alignment principles that teach proper posture and healthy body mechanics. Being strong, supple, and well aligned enhances your body's ability to meet the challenges of daily life with ease as well as its ability to release tension, improve circulation, and boost energy flow.

Breathing Practices: In a culture where people tend to be shallow "chest breathers," learning to breathe deeply and fully offers great physiological and psychological benefits. Bringing air down into the lowest portion of the lungs, where oxygen exchange is most efficient, triggers a cascade of changes: heart rate slows, blood pressure decreases, muscles relax, anxiety eases, and the mind calms. In contrast, chest breathing can lead to, or exacerbate, neck pain because it uses accessory respiratory muscles around the neck, such as the scalenes, to lift the chest, creating compression on the cervical spine (see chapter 2, figure 2.3, for an illustration of this area).

Mindfulness: Yoga is a practice of awareness that teaches us to be present in each moment and to be present in our bodies. This can be quite a challenge in our modern world, where people tend to live in the head while ignoring signals from the rest of the body to the extent that the body must scream in pain to get attention. Yoga counters this tendency to live from the neck up by helping us connect our minds and bodies through the breath. The practice invites us to bring our attention inward, recognize where we habitually hold tension, and learn to release it.

Meditation: Many of us tend to have chattering thoughts constantly rattling around in our heads: *What's next on my to-do list? Did I turn off the stove? I wonder what's on TV tonight?* This is a condition of chronic mental busyness that many meditation teachers call "monkey mind." Meditation is a powerful tool for calming the agitated mind, helping us to release distracting (and often anxiety-provoking) thoughts and to bring our attention and awareness to the present moment.

These varied tools work in a synergistic fashion. In his book, *Yoga as Medicine*, Dr. Timothy McCall (2007, 4) writes, "You stretch and strengthen your muscles, and that affects your circulation, digestion, and breathing. You calm and strengthen the nervous system, and it affects the mind. You cultivate peace of mind, and it affects the nervous system, the immune system, and the cardiovascular system. Yoga says that if you look clearly, you will see that everything about you is connected to everything else."

So it should come as no surprise to learn that yoga therapists don't just tell their clients, "Take this pose and call me in the morning." Practicing physical postures can be extremely beneficial in preventing and relieving neck pain and other ailments, but true healing involves both what you do on the mat and how you live your life. If the minute you leave your yoga mat, you begin to slump and tense your shoulders, you'll make less progress in relieving your neck pain than if you bring the teachings of yoga into your day-to-day activities. For example, paying attention to sitting and standing with good posture throughout your day; using a headset instead of holding the phone between your shoulder and ear; and taking slow, deep breaths whenever you feel stressed are basic ways to integrate yoga practice into your life.

Yoga also teaches that it's not just *what* you do, but *how* you do it that's critical. Unlike the Western exercise mentality that says the harder you work, the better the results, in yoga we often go deeper, not by *working harder* but by "playing softer," an inquisitive approach to the practice that cultivates the ability to relax, release, and let go. Yoga encourages you to balance effort and surrender, courage and caution—to challenge yourself but *never* strain. In yoga practice, learning how to "undo" is as important (and for some people *more* important) as learning how to "do." (See chapter 5, "How to Practice.") Rather than muscle your way into a yoga pose, you learn to relax into it—using the tools of gravity, patience, and the breath—to allow the pose to deepen and unfold.

Over time, with regular practice, the lessons learned on the yoga mat begin to influence how you live in the world. So when your boss comes charging into your office with an urgent assignment, instead of engaging in your habitual reaction of tensing your shoulders and gritting your teeth, you may find yourself responding by pausing to take a deep, slow breath and then consciously

> *Balance effort and surrender, courage and caution—challenge yourself but never strain. Learning how to "undo" is as important as learning how to "do."*

relaxing your shoulders. Or when turbulence begins to bounce the plane you're flying in, you may close your eyes, turn your attention to your breath, and begin lengthening your exhalations to calm your body and mind. Yoga teaches you how to relax and breathe as you bring yourself into challenging postures on the mat so that when you find yourself in challenging positions in daily life, you can draw on these skills to keep yourself balanced and healthy.

Exploring the Evidence

Western medical research into yoga's therapeutic benefits is relatively new, but it's booming—with more than a thousand studies involving yoga listed in the National Library of Medicine's research database, PubMed (www.ncbi.nlm.nih.gov/pubmed). Currently in the United States, more than sixty-five federally and privately supported clinical trials are under way examining yoga's benefits for a variety of conditions, including insomnia, heart failure, pediatric headaches, epilepsy, diabetes, obesity, hot flashes, arthritis, posttraumatic stress disorder, and cigarette addiction (ClinicalTrials. gov, www.clinicaltrials.gov, s.v., "Yoga"). And an emerging body of literature suggests that yoga can relieve a wide array of ailments, including chronic low-back pain, hypertension, irritable bowel syndrome, menopausal and perimenopausal symptoms, depression, anxiety, fibromyalgia, carpal tunnel syndrome, and obsessive-compulsive disorder. Yoga's effect on neck pain has not yet been the subject of published scientific study, but strong evidence for yoga's effectiveness in relieving back pain gives hope that research will eventually support yoga as effective self-care for neck pain as well (Sherman et al. 2005).

One clear benefit of yoga that most experts agree on is its ability to relieve stress, which is extremely important, since 60 to 90 percent of all doctor's office visits in the United States are stress related (Benson 1996). Stress has been shown to have wide-ranging effects on emotions, mood, and behavior. In her book, *Self-Nurture* (2000, 28), pioneering mind-body medicine expert Alice D. Domar notes that "chronic stress can trigger continually high levels of stress hormones (for example, adrenaline and cortisol) that produce elevated blood pressure or heart rate, increased oxygen consumption, weakened immune systems, and other physiologic imbalances that eventually lead to symptoms or even full-blown diseases." Domar calls yoga a "powerful approach...for relaxation and reinvigoration of mind and body" (42), and writes that many of her patients "report that yoga is among the most effective stress-relieving methods they've ever practiced" (112).

Therapeutic Yoga

Yoga is increasingly being used in modern medical settings as an adjunct therapy for a wide array of health concerns—from heart disease to hot flashes. Some pioneering medical centers (such as Duke Integrative Medicine, where I practice yoga therapy), clinics, and private studios offer individualized yoga sessions known as *yoga therapy*. In these one-on-one sessions, a yoga therapist adapts the practice to suit your specific needs, creating a personalized yoga program designed for practice at home. Typically, this involves yoga postures, breathing exercises, and relaxation techniques. Yoga therapy can be particularly helpful for people who are unable to participate in a regular group class or who have specific concerns, such as fibromyalgia, hypertension, or asthma. The goal of these sessions is to empower you to progress toward greater health and well-being.

In addition, a growing number of hospital-based wellness centers offer yoga classes for general well-being, as well as yoga classes designed for specific groups, such as breast cancer survivors; people with MS, heart disease, and chronic pain; and adolescents with eating disorders. Therapeutically oriented yoga classes are usually based on a gentle style of yoga. It's important to recognize that there are many different schools and kinds of yoga—including some that are quite challenging. For example, *Ashtanga* yoga is very athletic, while *Kripalu* yoga tends to be gentler.

It's fine to attend a yoga class to complement your practice with this book, as long as the class is appropriate for you and is taught by a well-trained and experienced yoga instructor. Unfortunately yoga's booming popularity has resulted in some classes that are called yoga but are actually "yoga-flavored" exercise classes taught by instructors whose training consists of attendance at a weekend yoga workshop. (See the resources section for help finding qualified yoga instruction.) If you attend a large group yoga class that's too demanding for your specific fitness level or one that's taught by a poorly trained or inexperienced instructor, you may risk injury. Ask prospective teachers how long they've taught yoga, where they studied, and, equally important, how long they've *practiced* yoga and whether or not they have a personal yoga practice. Authentic yoga instruction is rooted in a teacher's own yoga practice, and the best yoga teachers live their yoga on and off the mat. A skilled yoga instructor will *not* be a drill sergeant but will act as a facilitator—pointing you in the direction of your own "inner *guru*" (teacher) and helping you explore what works best for you.

the heart of the practice

Although yoga practices are designed to enhance our well-being, yogic tradition doesn't view improved health as an end in itself but, rather, as a quality necessary to properly connect with the spirit. The ancient yogis considered disease to be an obstacle to enlightenment. After all, it's difficult to sit still in meditation and unite with the divine if you have a pounding headache or a stiff neck. Likewise, if illness or sedentary habits have left you too weak and inflexible to sit comfortably, yoga postures and breathing practices can help you become healthy and strong enough to sit quietly and meditate. The body is considered a temple of the soul, and yoga practice helps maintain this precious vessel.

The focus of yoga practice is to quiet the mind. The *Yoga Sutras of Patanjali*, the ancient text that sets forth the teaching of yoga in 196 succinct aphorisms, states: "Yoga is the restriction of the fluctuations of consciousness."

Since a peaceful, stable mind is essential to well-being, the many tools of yoga are all designed to help calm the mind and harness its power for physical, psychological, emotional, and spiritual healing.

When the mind and body are peaceful, it's much easier to hear that "still, small voice" of the heart. Just as it's difficult to see the bottom of a lake when the air is agitated by wind— making the waters choppy and turbulent—it can be difficult to connect with our spirit when we're physically and emotionally restless. But when everything becomes calm and peaceful, we can see

> *"Yoga is the restriction of the fluctuations of consciousness."*

clearly to the bottom of the lake and to the innermost recesses of our heart.

In the yogic tradition, the spirit is often called our "true self" or "ultimate nature." These teachings hold that our spirits are alike— and that they're formless, immortal, and blissful. The familiar salutation, *Namaste*, a Sanskrit greeting typically said at the end of yoga class, translates—in short form—to "I honor you." But the more accurate explanation of this simple greeting is this:

> *I honor the place in you that is the same in me.*
> *I honor the place in you where the whole universe resides.*
> *I honor the place in you of love, light, truth, and peace.*
> *When you are in that place in you, and I am in that place*
>   *in me,*
> *We are one.*
> —Source unknown

Please be aware that, while yoga has a spiritual component, it's *not* a religion. You don't need to believe in any specific deity or even to believe in God at all to practice yoga. People of all faiths, as well as agnostics and atheists, are regular yoga practitioners. And it's fine to embrace those aspects of the practice that appeal to you and ignore the rest. Modifying the practice to suit your needs applies not just to postures but to the spiritual dimension as well.

how to use this book

If you're like many people, who think yoga is a kind of exercise, and you picked up this book to learn some "healing moves," hang in there. We offer dozens of illustrated postures in chapter 5, a detailed guide to proper sitting and standing posture in chapter 4, and a summarized "Neck Check" of easy, portable yoga practices to do on and off the mat in chapter 6.

By now I hope you understand that the profound healing available through yoga centers on uniting your body, mind, and spirit. Chapter 2 examines neck and shoulder pain from the perspective of the physical body—discussing anatomy, posture, and body mechanics—and offers insights into how the yoga practice can bring relief. Chapter 3 explores how emotions and stress influence neck pain, and offers the yogic perspective on the "energy body," with practical strategies you can use to learn how to identify and release habitual patterns of tension. Feel free to skip ahead to the postures and practice directions if you like, but be sure to come back to these foundational chapters for a comprehensive grounding in the yogic teachings, which will deepen your practice and enhance its healing power.

the inside story: anatomy, posture, & pain

If you've ever watched a toddler learn how to walk, you have a good idea of the delicate balancing act involved in keeping the heavy head poised atop the vertical spine. The neck is a slender conduit that connects the head to the torso, and it must be both strong and flexible to carry out the important task of supporting the skull with its precious cargo of brain and sensory organs. A complex structure, the neck is designed to allow the head to move in various directions to facilitate the work of the eyes, ears, nose, and mouth.

Whether you're engaged in a simple task, such as eating a meal, or a complicated maneuver, like hunting a wild boar, changing a tire, or dancing the tango, your neck may be required to bend forward, tilt sideways, arch back, turn right or left, or a combination of all these motions, sometimes in rapid succession. Even "doing nothing," such as just sitting and watching TV, can be tough on your neck because it must still support your head. It is the neck's flexibility, and its continual responsibility of holding up the heavy head, that exposes it to a wide array of stresses and strains.

Neck pain and associated tension often spreads to related body parts, such as the head, face, jaw, upper back, shoulders, and arms. Understanding some basic anatomy and becoming aware of our habitual postures and movement patterns can shed light on the causes of neck and shoulder pain, and offer strategies for lasting relief.

the spine

A column of cylindrical bones known as vertebrae, the human spine extends from the back of the head to the pelvis. Stacked on top of each other like a string of pearls, each vertebra has a solid part in front, called the *vertebral body*, and a space in the back that provides a protected passageway for the spinal cord. Together, the brain and spinal cord form the central nervous system, which coordinates the activity of all parts of the body.

In between each vertebra is a disc, a thick pad of cartilage with a jelly-like center that acts as a shock absorber and facilitates spinal movement. A complex system of muscles and ligaments holds everything in place.

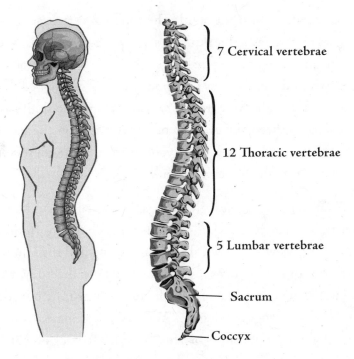

7 Cervical vertebrae

12 Thoracic vertebrae

5 Lumbar vertebrae

Sacrum

Coccyx

Figure 2.1. The Spine

The vertebrae change in size and shape, moving from larger bones at the bottom of the spine to smaller ones at the top. They're organized into four main regions:

Sacral: The sacrum is a triangular bone at the base of the vertebral column consisting of five fused, modified vertebrae. Attached to the tip of the sacrum is the *coccyx*, sometimes called the "tailbone."

Lumbar: Five lumbar vertebrae support the lower back.

Thoracic: Twelve thoracic vertebrae in the chest area connect to the body's ribs.

Cervical: Seven cervical vertebrae support the neck, with the two at the very top, C1 and C2, specialized for articulation with the skull. The topmost vertebra, C1, sits just underneath the skull and is nicknamed "atlas," after the mythological figure forced by Zeus to support the earth and heavens on his shoulders. C2 is dubbed "axis" because it's the axis around which C1 and the skull rotate when the head turns. That bump you feel on the back of your neck when you drop your chin to your chest is the lowest part of the cervical spine, C7.

Four natural curves give the spine strength and resilience, offering a springlike action that cushions the body from impact. From a side view, the cervical spine at the top and the lumbar spine at the bottom each curve toward the inside of the body, while the thoracic spine and sacral area each curve toward the outside.

A famous yogic saying is, "You are as young as your spine," honoring the importance of this central channel of our bodies. Much of the yoga practice is devoted to cultivating strength, flexibility, and proper alignment of this remarkable structure. In her comprehensive guide, *Yoga and You* (1996, 49), my teacher, Esther Myers, called the spine "the structural, nervous, and energy core of the body. It is the axis around which we can orient and through which we can ground. When we connect to our spines, we are connected to the core of who we are, where we stand, and what we believe and value."

Even our language appreciates this significance, calling a weak person "spineless" and admiring the integrity of someone with "backbone." To support us in moving efficiently and effectively through our busy days, our spine, in turn, needs our support in maintaining good posture and proper alignment. Unfortunately, in our sedentary society, poor posture is rampant.

postural stress

If you watch people as they walk, sit, or stand, you'll see why so many of us suffer from pain in the neck, shoulders, and back. While neck pain sometimes results from trauma, such as an injury from playing sports or whiplash from a car accident, by far the most common cause is stress on muscles and ligaments, often stemming from poor postural habits. Two major postural problems, which yoga can relieve and sometimes eliminate, are asymmetry and forward head.

Asymmetry

If you look at the soles of an old, favorite pair of walking shoes, you'll notice that they're likely to be worn in a particular pattern that reflects your repetitive habits of use. If your foot tends to roll in too much (overpronation), the shoe soles will be more worn down on the insides, and if your foot doesn't roll in enough (underpronation), they'll be more worn down on the outsides. Your physical structure can also reflect repetitive patterns of use so that, after years of using your muscles and ligaments in a specific way—often favoring one side of the body—you may become asymmetrical or lopsided. For example, one shoulder may be higher than the other or sit more forward than the other. Sometimes this asymmetry is linked to an inherent structural abnormality, such as scoliosis, which may be outside of your control. But often such an asymmetry is related to our repetitive habits of use, which in turn are frequently linked to our preference for using our dominant hand, for instance, the right-handed waiter who always carries trays on the left side to be able to distribute plates with the dominant hand. Other examples include:

- ✦ Carrying a heavy purse on one shoulder

- ✦ Holding a baby on one hip

- ✦ Cradling the telephone between the shoulder and the ear

- ✦ One-sided sports, such as golf, bowling, and tennis

- ✦ One-sided jobs, such as machine operator, concert violinist, and house painter

Over time, these kinds of repetitive patterns of use can lead to an imbalance in the body that's a setup for pain. For this reason, yoga practice is designed to help balance the body so that we become as symmetric as possible and all sides—right and left, front and back, top and bottom—have equal or appropriate strength and flexibility. Even for people with scoliosis or other structural abnormalities, yoga practice can be extremely therapeutic, helping to appropriately strengthen what's weak and lengthen what's short, thereby cultivating as much balance and symmetry throughout the body as possible.

Forward Head

Another common postural problem leading to neck pain is a misaligned relationship between the head and the shoulders, known as *forward head*, where the head protrudes in front of the shoulders and the upper back rounds. In our computerized, sedentary culture, forward head posture is rampant.

Consider this: almost everything we do throughout the day rounds our bodies forward. Whether we're working from a laptop or smartphone; working at a desk; performing manual labor like digging or sawing; or engaging in domestic activities like cooking, knitting, or rocking a baby, our focus is always forward and our bodies tend to round in response. With rare exceptions, such as painting a ceiling, almost nothing we do in our daily lives bends us backward.

The all-too-common result of spending so much time hunched over computers, steering wheels, and desks is this postural habit of holding the head in front of the shoulders. Often, the shoulders round forward too. In extreme cases, the chest also collapses and the chin juts out. Forward head posture is linked to a wide array of ailments, from headaches and stiff neck to breathing problems, digestive difficulties, and backache.

To understand why forward head posture leads to pain, look back at figure 2.1, which shows the healthy spine, and you'll see the head balanced directly over the shoulder girdle. From a side view, the hole in the ear lines up just over the shoulder. Think of that toddler who figured out how to position the head straight on top of the spine. When we're properly aligned like this, the skeleton can do its job of supporting the body with a minimum of muscular effort. In contrast, look at figure 2.2, which shows forward head posture, and notice how this postural misalignment forces our muscles, tendons, and ligaments to work overtime just to keep us from falling on our faces.

Remember, the head is heavy! The adult human head weighs roughly ten pounds, about the same as a bowling ball. Imagine holding a bowling ball in front of you all day, and you'll get a feel for what happens with forward head posture. When you carry your head in front of your shoulders, your neck and surrounding muscles must work extra hard to support its weight against the pull of gravity. This misalignment can compromise your shoulder joint, leading to inflammation in the surrounding tissues (tendinitis or

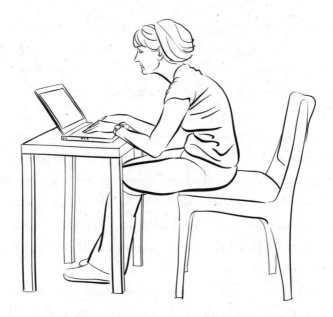

Figure 2.2. Forward-Head Posture

bursitis) and pain. Forward head posture can even adversely affect your lower back, since the curve in your lumbar spine (which supports your lower back) changes to offset the shift in your cervical spine.

This is why habitually sitting and standing with a forward head posture creates tension and strain in the neck, shoulders, and back, often leading to headaches and upper body pain. In addition, this "crunched" forward posture can interfere with proper breathing, circulation, and digestion. Once neck problems have developed, poor posture is likely to perpetuate them and frequently make them worse.

— Forward Head Self-Test —

The best way to determine whether or not you have forward head posture is to consult a physical therapist or experienced yoga teacher or yoga therapist. But you can also try one of these self-tests:

- *Up Against the Wall:* Stand with your back against a wall, with your heels touching the wall. If the back of your head doesn't easily touch the wall, you may have forward head.

- *Number One:* Make a fist and extend your index finger, as if you're signaling, "We're number one!" at a sports event. Keeping your hand in this position, place the base of your thumb against your sternum, right under your collarbone, so that your index finger is vertical, pointing toward the sky. If you have good posture, your chin will rest behind your extended finger. If your chin protrudes past your finger, you may have forward head posture and be at increased risk of neck pain.

the neck's neighbors: upper back, shoulders, jaw, and head

Neck pain is rarely isolated just to the neck region. Yoga makes us aware that everything is interconnected, so it's not surprising that nearby muscles and joints—in the upper back, shoulders, jaw, head, and face—may also experience discomfort. But many people don't realize that even seemingly unrelated issues, such as bunions on our feet or wearing high-heeled shoes, may contribute to poor posture that leads to neck pain. In addition, your overall fitness level can affect your ability to maintain good posture and "keep your head on straight." That's why yoga practice to heal neck and shoulder pain includes some general overall-conditioning postures (see chapter 5).

Here's a brief anatomical overview of areas above and below the neck that may affect, and be affected by, neck pain.

Shoulders and Upper Back

The shoulder area is where the arms meet the torso, and it involves several joints and a complex array of muscles, tendons, and ligaments designed to allow the arms to move through a wide range of motion. The main joint of the shoulder is the *glenohumeral joint*, which links the head of the major bone in the upper arm, the humerus, to the scapula. Also known as the shoulder blades, the scapulae lie in the back of the body near the rib cage, but are not attached to the ribs. Instead they're suspended by a network of muscles and ligaments that attach to the neck and upper spine, allowing them great mobility to rise up and down, to move away from and toward the spine, and to rotate.

34

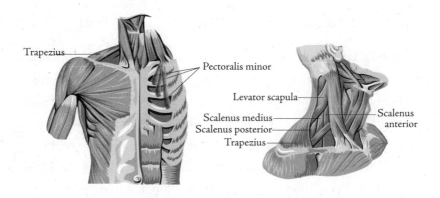

Figure 2.3. Muscles of the Neck and Shoulder Area

The shoulder girdle is formed by the humerus, scapula, and clavicle, also known as the collarbone. An intricate web of surface and deep muscles are involved in moving the neck, head, and shoulders. The muscles that often play a role in neck pain are:

- *Levator scapula*, extending from the cervical (neck) vertebrae to the inner-upper scapula (shoulder blade).

- *Trapezius*, extending from the base of the skull and the cervical and thoracic vertebrae, and inserting into the scapula and clavicle.

- *Pectoralis minor*, extending from ribs 3 to 5 and inserting into the top of the scapula.

- *Scalenes*, consisting of three muscles: *scalenus anterior* and *scalenus medius*, extending from the cervical spine and inserting into rib 1; and *scalenus posterior*, extending from the cervical spine and inserting into rib 2.

Face and Jaw

Our facial muscles get quite a workout from smiling, frowning, grimacing, scowling, and going through various other contortions throughout the day. Often these facial expressions are intentional and serve as a means of expressing who we are and how we feel. For example, think of the evil leer of Captain Hook, the broad grin of Bozo the Clown, or the peaceful countenance of the Dalai Lama. But in addition, many of us develop habitual patterns of expression that we may not even be aware of. For example, some common facial habits include furrowing the eyebrows or pursing the lips when concentrating. Those with poor eyesight may continually squint, often also pulling their heads forward as they strain to see. The mouth is often involved in facial habits, such as teeth grinding, lip pursing, tongue pressing, and cheek sucking.

Stress plays a strong role in habits that tense our facial muscles, which we'll explore more fully in chapter 3. But in becoming aware of our postural habits that can contribute to neck pain, it's important to recognize that all of our habitual patterns of use, including our facial expressions and stress reactions, may play a role in chronic neck pain.

A complex and poorly understood condition that's frequently associated with neck pain is *temporomandibular joint and muscle disorders* (TMJD), an ailment involving pain in and around the temporomandibular joint, which connects the lower jaw to the skull (Hampton 2008). Previously known as TMJ, the condition was renamed TMJD in 2004 by a coalition of federal health agencies because emerging research suggests it's much more than just a problem with the jaw joint. New evidence indicates that TMJD is actually a group of conditions rooted in a complex and interrelated web of genetic, psychological, environmental, and biological causes.

Neck pain is common among people with TMJD, which is also associated with headaches, earaches, and teeth grinding.

To feel your temporomandibular joint (also known as TMJ) at work, place your fingers just in front of your ears, and open and close your mouth a few times. The "bumps" you feel are the rounded ends of the lower jaw, called *condyles*, gliding along the joint socket of the temporal bone on the side of the head. The TMJ is our body's most highly used joint, and also one of the most complicated. It combines both sliding and hinging motions to allow the jaw to move side to side, up and down, and front to back. Many of life's most exciting and enjoyable activities depend on a well-functioning TMJ, for example, kissing, chewing, singing, swallowing, biting, and carrying on a conversation. Adding to the complexity is the need for both TMJ joints to work as a team. So it's not surprising that these small joints are frequently the location of major—and sometimes devastating—pain.

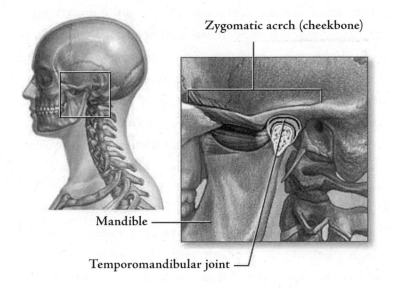

Figure 2.4. TMJD

Presently there's no widely accepted, standard test available to diagnose the disorder. In most cases, the patient's description of symptoms, a physical examination of the face and jaw, and a detailed medical and dental history are used. While traditionally dentists have treated TMJD, it's not uncommon for frustrated and sometimes desperate patients to see multiple health care providers in their search for answers, including neurologists, rheumatologists, sleep specialists, and chiropractors. Emerging research suggests that TMJD is a pain condition that responds well to self-care practices—including yoga and relaxation training—that teach you to breathe correctly, stretch tight muscles, and learn to release tension from painful places throughout your body.

coming out of a slump

One of the biggest challenges in learning to "undo" chronic tension and regain healthy, balanced alignment is that most of our postural habits are deeply ingrained. So these are not problems that will go away overnight. Proper posture is something you need to be aware of continually throughout the day. (See chapter 6 for yoga "micro-practices" to integrate into your life.) And posture is also something to be mindful of at night. If you've ever woken up with a stiff neck, you're well aware that sleeping with poor posture can contribute to neck and shoulder pain. (See chapter 4 for guidelines on healthy sleeping alignment.)

With regular practice and patience, over time you'll make substantial progress. While improving posture takes work, the results—pain relief, improved health, and enhanced appearance—can be far reaching. One unexpected bonus is the "instant weight loss" effect of good posture. Slumping can cause the belly to protrude, which means that when you learn how to stand properly, it can look as if you've suddenly lost five pounds.

> *Everything is interconnected.*

In addition, good posture can give you an emotional lift, since the way you hold your body affects the way you feel, and vice versa. People who carry themselves with good alignment seem confident and graceful, while those whose posture reflects a physical slump often appear to be in a mental slump as well.

This relationship between our physical posture and our emotional state reinforces the yogic wisdom that everything is interconnected. We'll explore the connection between our emotions and our neck and shoulder pain in the next chapter.

the emotional connection: the role of stress & the energetic body in neck & shoulder pain

Suppose you switch on the radio and hear that:

- A category 5 hurricane is headed toward your city.

- Your employer is in financial trouble and will be laying off staff.

- Health officials have closed your child's school because it houses a dangerous mold.

- The government has raised the terror alert to red for "severe risk" of attacks.

Can you feel the sense of alarm such unsettling news can cause? Do you notice how *mental* distress tends to manifest itself in your *physical* body? Perhaps your brow furrows, your muscles tense, and your breath quickens. You may even feel "butterflies" in your stomach.

Humans are hardwired with this mind-body link so that our perception of danger prompts physiological responses designed for self-preservation. In infants, numerous survival reflexes are apparent, including the startle reflex, instantly pulling the arms and legs inward after a loud noise, and the grasp reflex, when a baby's hand closes around a finger placed on her open palm. Pediatricians typically test newborns to make sure they respond appropriately to specific stimuli, since the absence of certain involuntary muscle reactions may suggest damage to the brain or nervous system. Infant reflexes normally disappear with age, but some reflexes persist into adulthood, including the gag reflex, when the throat or back of the mouth is stimulated, and the sneeze reflex, when your nasal passages are irritated. And we continue to have startle reactions to surprising stimuli, such as loud noises and bright lights.

Think about your own response to an explosive thunderclap, or even to someone's sneaking up behind you and saying, "Boo!"

the stress response

Nature has equipped us with a brilliantly coordinated "fight-or-flight" reaction designed to help us do battle or flee when we're in harm's way. When faced with danger, the body releases adrenaline and other hormones into the bloodstream, prompting a cascade of physiological changes—including speeding up the heart rate and tensing muscles—to boost our ability to react to an emergency. This is extremely useful if we're running for our lives from a tiger: the body revs up to fight or flee, then ratchets back down when the crisis is over. But in our modern world, stress is more likely to come from chronic pressures (such as financial worries and work deadlines) that are relentless, leaving many people in a state of hyperarousal or permanent fight or flight, with these physiological changes stuck in emergency mode. Over time, chronic stress can weaken the immune system and increase the risk of numerous ailments, including heart disease, heart attack, and stroke.

Western medical science began recognizing the health hazards of chronic stress and the importance of turning off the fight-or-flight response in the 1970s, when Harvard-trained cardiologist Dr. Herbert Benson coined the term "relaxation response" to describe the beneficial changes associated with deep meditation, including reduced heart rate and blood pressure, slower breathing, and decreased muscle tension. Research by Dr. Benson and his colleagues showed that eliciting the relaxation response can counter the harmful effects of chronic stress (Benson 1996). Over the last several decades, a growing body of scientific evidence supports the health benefits of regularly calming the body and mind through various techniques, including meditation, guided imagery, and yoga. Yoga is a particularly effective mind-body practice that appears to enhance stress-coping mechanisms, according to the National Center for Complementary and Alternative Medicine, which is funding research to investigate yoga's effects on a variety of stress-related ailments, including insomnia, smoking cessation, and post-traumatic stress disorder (NCCAM 2008).

Although the harmful effects of chronic stress are now well documented, evidence suggests that, unfortunately, our lives are becoming increasingly stressful. More than 50 percent of adults in the United States report high stress on a daily basis, according to the Benson-Henry Institute for Mind Body Medicine at Massachusetts General Hospital (www.massgeneral.org/bhi/basics/stress.aspx). And in the United Kingdom, a 2009 report by the Mental Health Foundation, called "In the Face of Fear," revealed that 1 in 7 adults has anxiety disorders, 800,000 more than in the early nineties. More than a third (37 percent) said they feel more frightened than they used to, and a majority (77 percent) thinks the world has become more frightening in the last ten years (Mental Health Foundation 2009).

Pain in the Neck from the Weight of the World on Your Shoulders

Just as postural habits, such as forward head, can contribute to neck and shoulder pain (see chapter 2), our psychobiological habits, how we respond emotionally and physically to stress, may also play an important role. For example, when we're faced with fear, anxiety, or other stressors, one of the most common reactions is to tighten muscles in the upper back, shoulders, and neck—in effect, lifting the shoulders up toward the ears. It's almost as if we're trying to protect our heads the way a turtle draws its head and limbs into its shell. Other common reactions to stress that involve the neck and shoulders include teeth grinding, lip pursing, and other facial grimaces, along with finger drumming, thumb twiddling, and various forms of fidgeting.

Over time, these physical responses to stress can become habitual patterns so that we develop a kind of rigid "body armor" of tight, overused muscles in the neck and shoulders. When stress is chronic, these muscles may stay tense and never, or rarely, let go. Often this pattern becomes so ingrained that we don't even notice we're holding tension.

This connection between emotional distress and pain in the neck and shoulders is so common that our culture has created the phrase "a pain in the neck" to describe a stressful situation or an unpleasant person. And it's no surprise that we describe the feeling of being under intense pressure as having "the weight of the world" on our shoulders. Clearly our emotions can have a profound effect on our bodies: how we carry ourselves, where we hold tension, and how we experience pain.

Awareness of this problem is the first step in learning to let it go. One of my yoga students has developed the simple mantra *Relax your shoulders*, which she frequently recites mentally to herself, for example, if she's having trouble sleeping or when she's stuck in traffic or waiting in line. "I never realized how much tension I hold in my shoulders," she told me. "But whenever I consciously think about it, I realize that my shoulders are up around my ears. When I take a deep breath and invite my shoulders to relax, everything softens and lets go."

—— Awareness Practice: ——
Recognizing Habitual Patterns of Tension

Habits are typically mindless behaviors, actions we take without thinking, such as chewing our fingernails in response to stress. As a practice of awareness, yoga helps shine light on these often-unconscious links between emotional and physical stress. In yoga, we use our breath to bring us into the present moment and also to connect the body with the mind. Yoga helps us counter the tendency to live "from the neck up" and encourages us to pay attention to what's happening throughout our entire being—physically, emotionally, energetically, and spiritually.

California yoga teacher and physical therapist Judith Hanson Lasater offered this wonderful analogy for how yoga works when I interviewed her for a *Prevention* magazine article: "Yoga is like a speed bump that slows you down so you pay attention to your body" (Lasater 2004). Most of us can relate to this connection between mindless driving and mindless living. If you've ever pulled into the parking lot at a familiar destination and then realized you barely remember how you got there, you know how easy it is to do important, and even dangerous, things in a mindless manner. But the "speed bump" of yoga practice gets our attention and encourages us to be present and notice what's happening in our lives—right now in this moment.

The following five-step yogic awareness practice is designed to help you tease out the ways your body responds to stress and where you tend to experience and store tension, plus potentially uncover the emotional connections to your physical discomforts. Please approach this practice mindfully, in a nonjudgmental spirit of self-exploration and self-discovery, with compassion and kindness for yourself. You might want to imagine that you're a curious and persistent detective, looking for clues and connections to unlock the mysteries of your neck and shoulder pain.

1. **Tuning In:** Lie down on your back or recline in a chair in a way that makes you feel comfortable and supported. Arrange your body to be as symmetrical as possible so that, if there were a line bisecting you from nose to navel, your right and left sides would be equidistant from that line. Close your eyes if you like, or keep them open with a soft gaze. (Be sure that you've eliminated distractions: turn off your phone and ask family members not to disturb you.) Bring your attention to your breath and observe the sensations that occur as you breathe in and out.

2. **Body Scan A:** Now the detective work begins. With your mind's eye, take a journey throughout your interior landscape, looking for any places of tension or tightness, pain, discomfort, or "dis-ease." Pay particular attention to your upper body—neck, shoulders, arms, chest, and back—and see if any body parts are "talking" to you. If you find a tense area, try your best to describe the sensation: is it sharp or dull, achy or sore—knotty, warm, or grabby? If you feel pain, how intense is it on a scale of 1 to 10, with 1 being mild and 10 being severe? Are you experiencing more than one place of discomfort? If

so, do all the places feel similar, or are some areas more painful than others? Do these painful areas appear connected or disconnected? Make a mental note of any discoveries. Then see if you can relax and release any tense places, imagining your breath moving through the tight areas and helping them soften and let go.

3. **Recalled Event:** When you're ready, bring to mind an event in your life that you found distressing. Pick a real memory of a stressful situation. You might prefer to start with a mild annoyance, such as finding the post office closed when you needed to mail a package. Or you can choose something that was extremely upsetting, such as a bad day at work or an argument with a loved one. Recall the situation in as vivid detail as possible: What time of day did it occur? Who was there? What words were said? What gestures were made? Engage your senses so that you hear the voices, feel the textures, and even smell the aromas surrounding this difficult memory.

4. **Body Scan B:** As you mentally relive this stressful event, do another body scan, paying exquisite attention to the physical and emotional sensations that arise. What happens in your face, neck, mouth, shoulders, back, and belly? What happens to your breath? Does it quicken, or does it stop? What happens in your mind and in your heart? If you find one or more tense

areas, try your best to describe the sensations. If you feel pain, how intense is it? Is there more than one place of discomfort? If so, do they all feel similar, or are some areas more painful than others? Do they appear connected or disconnected? Make a mental note of any discoveries. Then see if you can relax and release any tense places, imagining your breath moving through the tight areas, helping them soften and let go.

5. **Journal:** When you're ready, open your eyes, take out a notebook, and write down what you've discovered. Remember, you're a sleuth looking for clues and connections, so write down all your observations of how you respond to stress, where you tend to experience and store tension, and any emotional connections to your physical discomforts. You may wish to keep making notes in this journal about how you respond to stress and any other mind-body links you discover over time as a result of your yoga practice.

Please recognize that the stress you may have experienced during this practice arose from stories happening in your mind. Despite your body's stress reactions, you were not in any real danger. As my Duke Integrative Medicine colleague Dr. Jeffrey Brantley notes in his excellent guide, *Calming Your Anxious Mind*, "Physical experience is deeply interconnected with psychological and emotional experience moment by moment. Physical sensations can trigger thoughts (such as when you perceive pain in your knee as arthritis and begin to think of the story of your arthritis and your fear of arthritis), and thoughts can stimulate physical responses (such as when you recall an angry outburst in a meeting, and your neck and shoulders immediately tense up)" (Brantley 2007, 13–14).

You may wish to try this practice again with different memories, exploring your reactions to a range of stressful events and using this exercise as a tool to understand your individualized stress response. In addition, consider using this "speed bump" practice whenever you find yourself in a stressful situation so that you slow down and notice what's happening. For example, you might use as "cues" any particular habits you recognize as your own signals of stress, such as chewing your lip, gritting your teeth, or holding your breath. When you feel these stress reactions occurring, pay attention to what's going on for you physically, emotionally, energetically, and spiritually. Unlocking the mysteries of your own habitual patterns of responding to stress is the first step in learning to let go of tension and make positive changes toward healing.

yogic perspective on pain and healing

Although Western medical science has only recently begun to explore the mind-body connection, the idea that thoughts and emotions play a powerful role in our health is an essential part of Eastern healing traditions. Both traditional Chinese medicine (TCM) and *Ayurveda* (traditional Indian medicine) recognize the importance of an intangible "vital energy" or "life force" that animates human beings. While there's no one word in English to describe this concept, it's known as *chi* in TCM, and *prana* in

Ayurveda, which is considered a "sister science" to yoga. Both of these disciplines consider the proper flow of this vital energy essential to health, and view disease as related to a blockage or other problem with the flow of chi or prana. Negative thoughts and emotions can weaken this flow, while positive thoughts and emotions can enhance it.

Prana is just one way in which the yogic view of human physiology differs from the Western model. Yogic teachings present a holistic view of the human being that takes into account much more than just muscles and bones but, rather, embraces the subtle energies of our lives that can profoundly impact our health. Ancient yoga texts describe your physical body as just the outermost layer of five bodies covering your true self, your inner light or spirit, which is the only unchanging part of your being. Often described as similar to Russian wooden dolls that nest one inside the other, these five bodies are known as *koshas* (sheaths). Listed in order of outermost to innermost, they are:

- *Annamaya Kosha: Anna* means "food" and represents the physical body, which is sustained by food from the earth. This outermost sheath is considered the "gross" body, because it's the part of ourselves we can feel, see, smell, and touch.

- *Pranamaya Kosha: Prana* means "energy body" and is the first of the three "subtle bodies" that can't be seen or touched but can be felt. As we breathe, we inhale prana, or life force, and yogic breathing practices, known as *pranayama*, are designed to enhance and cultivate this energy body. Like the gas that fuels the car, prana powers our physical bodies.

- *Manomaya Kosha:* This is the body of the mind and senses, sometimes called the "emotional body" because it houses our habitual patterns of thought and emotion. This layer houses our likes and dislikes, everything we've learned and perceived, even past slights and emotional "scars."

- *Vijnanamaya Kosha: Vijnana* means "knowing," and this is the body of higher wisdom, sometimes thought of as insight or discernment. Often experienced as a subjective witness speaking with a wise inner voice, this place of deep knowing can be challenging to reach. Gaining access to this layer of our being is a central part of spiritual practice.

- *Anandamaya Kosha: Ananda* means "bliss" or "joy," and is described as a feeling of unconditional love, wholeness, and integration. Called the "causal body," this kosha is considered the thinnest sheath or veil covering your true self, which is complete, whole, and blissful.

This yogic concept that human beings are comprised of multilayered gross and subtle bodies is based on the premise that body and mind are different but interrelated expressions of energy. Yoga practice is designed to enhance the flow of prana throughout all the pathways of the body and mind. These subtle energy channels are called *nadis* (channels), and there are generally said to be about seventy-two thousand of these energy pathways. Like water through a hose, energy flows through these nadis to sustain human life. But just as a kink in a hose will block the steady flow of water, blockage in a nadi—for example, from physical or emotional tension—is said to impede the flow of prana, which can lead to pain and disease.

the neck's challenge: connecting head and heart

From this yogic perspective, it's easy to see why the neck and shoulders are often a hot spot of chronic tension and pain. As the central channel connecting the head to the heart, the neck and shoulder region can be a bottleneck for emotional conflicts and spiritual struggles between what we think and what we feel. In her book, *The Healing Path of Yoga* (2000, 148–49), renowned yoga teacher Nischala Joy Devi writes, "...the neck is a superhighway passing messages from the head to the heart and the heart to the head. When the head and heart agree, the neck is like an open freeway, moving energy along at sixty miles per hour. If the head and the heart are at odds, the freeway gets jammed and the neck starts to ache. Ideally our hearts and minds will have equal input so we can make balanced decisions. The neck is then free from tension."

The heavy mental burdens many of us carry can also create tension and pain in the neck and shoulders, according to Devi (2000), who also states that chronic hunching can be a way to try to protect our hearts from emotional pain. "We are protecting them so much that we stop the love from flowing in and out," she writes (149). "As we relax our shoulders, we can lay down our burdens, and our chest and heart are able to expand."

Another factor that may contribute to the subtle body's relationship to neck pain is that, according to yogic tradition, the throat is the location of the *vishuddha chakra* (energy center of communication). The word *chakra* means "wheel," and each chakra is said to be a kind of spinning wheel or vortex of energy. Seven main chakras are located along the spine, from base to crown:

- *Muladhara* at the pelvic floor

- *Svadhishthana* at the pelvic basin

- *Manipura* at the solar plexus

- *Anahata* at the heart

- *Vishuddha* at the throat

- *Ajna* at the third eye (between the brows)

- *Sahasrara* at the crown of the head

Each chakra corresponds to particular physical, mental, and energetic aspects of our being. For example, the chakras in the lower body relate to more earthly concerns—such as material security (muladhara), sexuality and creativity (svadhishthana), and personal power (manipura)—while the chakras in the upper body relate to more spiritual areas, such as love and compassion (anahata), intuition (ajna), and enlightenment (sahasrara).

The throat chakra (vishuddha) is a center of communication, associated with expressing yourself honestly and clearly speaking your truth. Conflicts between what we think and what we say—for example, if we lie or repress anger—are thought to lead to pain or disease in this area. If you've ever experienced a "lump" in your throat, you may appreciate this yogic view of how turbulent thoughts and emotions can express themselves physically.

While there's no hard evidence supporting the existence of yogic concepts such as prana, koshas, and chakras, they're part of a five-thousand-year-old tradition that has sustained millions of people. Modern medicine is just beginning to turn its scientific inquiry to the health benefits of this ancient practice, and may unlock some of its mysteries. So, for now I invite you to simply consider these yogic notions and how they might relate to your own life. As always, take what works for you and leave the rest.

putting your head on straight: posture guidelines for daily life

One of the simplest and most effective ways to relieve, and hopefully eliminate, neck and shoulder pain is to improve your posture. But if you're like many people, posture is something you never think about. In fact, it's common for people to be totally unaware of their own habitual tendencies to stand and sit with poor alignment, not recognizing the connection between poor posture and pain. And even if you *do* know that your posture could use some improvement (perhaps your mother continually nagged you to "Stand up straight"), you may not know specifically what to do to correct your alignment.

This is why, when I give talks about yoga and health, I tell the audience, "Freeze. Stay exactly as you are. Don't move. Please take this time to notice how you're sitting." Typically there's some uncomfortable shuffling and, despite my admonition not to move, some surreptitious uncrossing of legs and straightening of spines. My motive isn't to embarrass people, but to get them to pay attention to their posture so they can make healthy changes. Then I offer some simple cues for ways to improve posture in virtually any situation.

So perhaps you've guessed what's coming next. I'd like you to do the same: Freeze. Stay exactly as you are. Don't move. Please take this time to notice how you're sitting. In particular, notice:

+ Where is your head in relationship to your shoulders? Is it sitting forward of your shoulder girdle or balanced on top of your spine?

+ What are you sitting on? Your "sit bones"? Your sacrum?

+ What shape is your spine? Are you slumped forward in a "C" shape, or is your spine long, maintaining its natural "S"-shaped curves?

+ Are your collarbones broad, or are they rounded forward?

+ Is your jaw clenched or relaxed? Are your teeth together or slightly apart? Is your tongue resting lightly in your mouth or pressed against your palate?

- Are your shoulders relaxed, down away from your ears, or are they tensed and lifted?

- Is your face relaxed, or are your brows furrowed, your lips pursed, or both?

- Is your chin tipped up, tucked down, or parallel to the ground?

- If an arrow came out of the top of your head, where would it point? Straight up or at a diagonal?

- Are you holding tension anywhere in your body? Do a quick body scan, looking for any places where you might be holding tension or tightness. (In addition to the face, neck, and shoulders, other common places to hold tension include the back, hands, and feet.) If you do discover that you're holding tension or tightness anywhere, take a deep abdominal breath (see chapter 5) and invite your exhalation to help you release any tension you feel.

I encourage you to do this simple practice throughout your day, taking a moment to briefly "freeze" and notice your posture. You might even set your watch or cell phone to chime or sound a "bell" every hour as a reminder to do this posture check. Whenever you hear the bell, pause and bring your attention to your posture, particularly noticing how your spine is positioned and the relationship of your head to your shoulders. Then use the practices outlined in this chapter to bring yourself into healthy alignment.

Simply becoming aware of your own postural habits is the first step to making important changes that can lead to lasting relief of neck and shoulder pain. To learn how to replace poor alignment habits with healthy ones, we'll explore how to have good posture throughout your day, whether you're standing, sitting, working at the computer, carrying groceries, or walking the dog. Read on to learn how to put your head on straight and "take a load off" your neck and shoulders.

standing on your own two feet

Our ability to stand upright on two legs is fundamental to our evolution as human beings. Standing with good alignment offers stability, helps us radiate confidence, and enhances our ability to use all of our limbs and to move through the world with ease. The yoga posture that teaches us proper standing alignment is called *tadasana*, which means "mountain pose." When properly executed, this posture helps us feel as strong and as stable as a mountain.

You'll find a detailed description and illustration of mountain pose in chapter 5 that will bring you into good standing alignment. But here, in this posture section, we'll explore how to bring this pose off the mat and into everyday life, with a few simple steps designed to help you find and maintain good posture anytime you're standing—whether you're moving or still.

The yogic perspective builds all postures from the foundation up, starting with whatever part of the body is connected to the earth. Depending on the pose, this could be almost any body part, from your hands to your head to your belly. But when we're standing up, of course, it's our feet that form the foundation of our posture. That's why it's critical to wear shoes that allow us to connect the entire foot to the earth and provide as broad a base of support as possible to maximize stability and skeletal health. Stiletto heels may be fashionable, but they throw off your posture by forcing you to balance on the balls of your feet, which distorts the natural curves of the spine.

In yoga, we sometimes imagine our feet as little cars, each of which has four wheels: one at the inner heel, one at the outer heel, one at the base of the big toe, and one at the base of the little toe. For proper standing posture, we press down evenly through each of these four "wheels" of our feet and lift up through the arches. The two rear "wheels" generally bear most of our body weight, since our heels are designed for this purpose. So clearly, it's critical to wear shoes that allow our heels to do their job. Shoes with small heels can be fine, as long as they're low enough to allow you to bring your body weight into your heels and feel the connection of all four "wheels" of your feet to the earth.

Here are eight simple steps to standing with good alignment:

1. Bring your feet hip-width apart, with your weight evenly distributed on both legs. Take a moment to feel the connection between the soles of your feet and the earth, and press down evenly through all four "wheels" of your feet. Become aware of your weight dropping down through your legs to your feet. Notice the contact of your heels with the floor, and imagine yourself growing roots through your entire foot so that you feel grounded and stable. Keep your breath slow, deep, and easy; avoid holding your breath.

2. Take one hand and gently pat yourself on the top of your head for a few moments, then relax your arm down by your side. Notice the sensation on the top of your head from the tapping; this is the crown of your head (for a review of the crown chakra, sahasrara, see chapter 3). You won't find this body part in *Gray's*

Anatomy, but the crown is very important in enhancing posture since extending this part of your head toward the sky helps lengthen your spine and bring the skull into alignment over the shoulder girdle. To help find this position, imagine that the crown of your head is magnetic and the ceiling is a powerful magnet, drawing the top of your head upward. Be sure to stay grounded through your feet as you lengthen up from your crown, so that your spine elongates and your head lifts up over your shoulder girdle.

3. Keep your chin parallel to the earth; avoid the common tendency to lift the chin up, which can "crunch" the back of your neck. It may help to also think of lifting up from the tops of your ears so that your neck lengthens.

4. Relax your shoulders down away from your ears, and invite your arms to relax comfortably at your sides.

5. Soften your knees so that your legs are straight but your knees aren't locked. Avoid hyperextending your knees, since this can lead to a swayback posture.

6. As you continue to root yourself down through your feet and lift up through the crown of your head, see if you can "stack your joints" so that if someone looked at you from the side, they'd see your knees over your ankles, your hips over your knees, your shoulders over your hips, and the little hole in your ear over your shoulder.

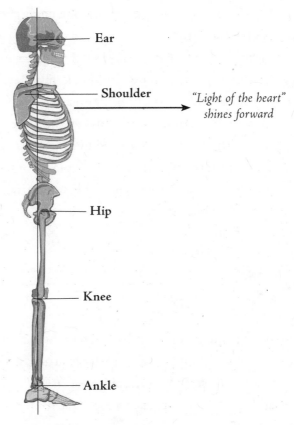

Ear

Shoulder

"Light of the heart" shines forward

Hip

Knee

Ankle

Figure 4.1. Stacked Joints

7. Gently draw your lower belly in and up, to support your lower back. Don't "suck in" your gut, or create any tension or hardness in your abdominal muscles. Just bring a little tone to this region by lightly engaging your abdominals, drawing your navel toward your spine.

8. Imagine that you have a light shining out from the center of your chest at your breastbone, the location of the heart chakra, anahata (see chapter 3 for review). Keep this light shining forward, not down toward the ground.

At first, coming into good alignment might seem difficult, if your body is used to bad habits such as standing with one hip slung out or the chest collapsed. But over time and with practice (including regular yoga to strengthen weak muscles and stretch tight ones), proper posture will become easier and virtually effortless. Standing with good alignment allows the skeleton to do its job in supporting the body with a minimum of muscular effort. And as you learn to bring your awareness to places of chronic tension and invite your breath to help you release any tightness, these good habits will become second nature, allowing you ease of movement and relief from pain.

sitting pretty

The basic principles of good sitting alignment are similar to those for proper standing posture. In fact, sitting with good alignment is often called "seated mountain pose" (see chapter 5). As with all postures, the yogic approach is to start from the foundation, with whatever part of our body supports us, and get grounded there. Then we extend away from that place of grounding, creating length in the spine.

When you're sitting in a chair, most of your weight rests on your bottom, with some on your feet. The parts of your pelvis meant to support you when you're sitting are the two rounded knobs at the base called the *ischial tuberosities*, better known (not surprisingly) as the "sit bones." Before the days of padded chairs, people naturally sat on their sit bones, since leaning back on the tailbone is very uncomfortable when you're on a hard surface. But in a world of upholstered chairs, cushy sofas, and plump pillows designed for lounging, reading, and watching TV in bed, many of us have lost touch with our natural sit bones and, instead, sit on the tailbone or sacrum, which is a setup for pain since this rounds the back and typically collapses the shoulders and juts the head forward.

Here are three simple steps to sitting on a chair with good alignment:

1. Place your feet flat on the floor. If they don't comfortably reach the floor, place them on a footstool.

2. Reach your hands under your bottom and feel for the two hard knobs at the base of your pelvis; these are your sit bones. Gently move the flesh of your buttocks aside so you can feel your sit bones releasing down onto the chair seat. Take a moment to get grounded; root down through your sit bones and feel the soles of your feet connect with the floor or footstool.

3. From this place of grounding, extend the crown of your head toward the sky, creating length in the spine. As with standing posture:

   a. Be sure to keep the chin parallel to the floor (avoid the tendency to tilt the chin up).

   b. Relax your shoulders down away from your ears.

   c. Imagine a light at your breastbone, and shine this "heart light" forward, not down toward the floor.

   d. Stack your joints so that if someone looked at you from the side, they'd see your shoulder directly over your hips and the hole in your ear directly over your shoulder.

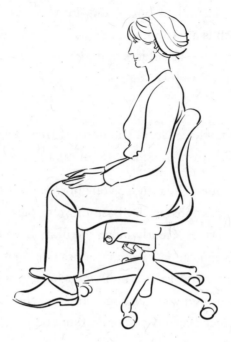

Figure 4.2. Sitting Pretty

proper posture in daily life

Three basic concepts will help you find good posture in virtually any situation:

+ Lengthen your spine and maintain its natural curves.

+ Keep your neck in line with your spine.

+ Use only the muscles you need, and relax the others.

Good posture is this simple. But in our stressful world, where many of us sit for extended periods—often in chairs designed for appearance or economy rather than postural support—finding and maintaining healthy alignment typically requires adjusting our environment so that it properly supports us. Here are some guide-lines to make sure you get the support you need:

At Your Desk: Be sure your chair fits your body and has a lumbar support to maintain the natural curves of your back. If your chair doesn't have good lumbar support, place a rolled towel or small pillow between your lower back and the chair. If your feet don't rest flat on the floor, use a footrest. Some new ergonomic chairs also come with a neck rest, which can be an excellent option to maintain the proper position of your head and avoid neck strain. If you use a laptop, consider using a docking station and an external monitor and keyboard to avoid crunching your body forward to see the screen. (The National Institutes of Health offers excellent advice on ergonomics for computer workstations at http://dohs. ors.od.nih.gov/ergo_computers.htm.) Avoid sitting for extended periods. Take brief walking breaks as often as possible, or at least stand up and stretch frequently, preferably for a few minutes every hour. In particular, arch your body back to counter the amount of time your body is focused forward (see seated back bend in chapter 5). Be aware, too, that intense focus on a computer screen tends to shut down the breath. Try to both sense and hear your breath when you're touching your keyboard, mouse, or both.

Grooming: Avoid rounding your body forward when brushing your teeth. Keep your spine long as you brush, then bend your knees and hinge forward from your hip joint (not your waist)— keeping length in your spine—when it's time to spit. Arrange your mirror so that you can keep your spine long, with its natural curves, when you're shaving or putting on makeup.

On the Phone: *Never* squeeze the receiver between your ear and shoulder; get in the habit of using a headset. (Inexpensive models that will plug into most cordless phones are available at popular electronics retailers.) Not only does this help you maintain good posture, but you'll also have both hands free and be able to use "phone time" to do some simple stretches.

Walking: Remember to lengthen up from the crown of your head and keep the light of your heart shining forward—not down in the gutter. Gaze forward, not down. If you must carry something heavy, use a backpack to distribute weight evenly across the body. But don't overload the backpack. If you need to carry something that weighs more than 10 to 15 percent of your body weight, consider a wheeled pack or suitcase and alternate which hand you use to pull it.

Sleeping: Consider sleeping on your back or side rather than on your stomach. Be sure your pillow supports the natural curve of your neck and doesn't prop your head up so high that your neck flattens. Choose a pillow made of a material that will conform to the shape of your neck, such as down.

In the Kitchen: During any standing activity—for example, washing lettuce, chopping vegetables, or stirring a pot—bring your awareness to your posture. Stand tall as you work and try to keep your shoulders relaxed and down away from your ears as you use your arms to cook.

Driving: Adjust your seat to allow your legs to move freely to reach the pedals while your back remains snug against the seat back. If your driver's seat doesn't have good lumbar support, consider purchasing a lumbar roll designed for this purpose, or place a small pillow between the small of your back and the seat. Make sure your mirrors are properly adjusted, and remember to keep your spine long (extending up from the crown) whenever you need to turn your head, for example, to change lanes. Use both of your hands on the steering wheel with a light grip, not a death grip, and relaxed shoulders. Ideally, for protection against whiplash in the event of an accident, the top of your head restraint should be at least as high as your head's center of gravity (or about three-and-a-half inches below the top of your head), with as little distance as possible from the back of your head to the restraint (preferably less than four inches), according to the Insurance Institute for Highway Safety (2009). Unfortunately not all cars are designed to make this possible. On long drives, take regular breaks to walk around and stretch.

In the Yard: Attention to posture can help you avoid pain, particularly during bending and lifting. Avoid rounding your back as you bend forward. Instead, bend your knees and hinge from your hip joint (not your waist) so that your spine stays long and maintains its natural curves. Keep objects that you're lifting as close to the middle of your body as possible. And remember to keep your neck in line with your spine.

Lounging Around: Whether you're snuggled on a couch, loveseat, or your favorite recliner, be sure that you're sitting on your sit bones, not your sacrum. It's fine to raise your feet on an ottoman; just be sure your back is comfortably supported (with pillows, rolled towels, or blankets if necessary) so that your spine is long and maintains its natural curves.

posture pointers

Simply being aware of your posture, doing your best to lengthen your spine and keep your head on straight, can have a profound effect on your neck and shoulder health. As part of this awareness practice, pay attention to your habitual patterns of using your body and notice how this affects your posture. For example, do you carry a heavy briefcase or shoulder bag that makes it difficult to maintain good posture? If so, consider other options, such as switching to a backpack, rolling bag, or even two smaller bags, holding one in each hand. Do you use only your dominant hand in activities of daily life? If so, play with using your nondominant hand to open doors, lift objects, wipe counters, or stir pots. Perhaps switch your computer mouse to the opposite side for a day and notice if you feel a difference in your neck and shoulders. A little "detective work," observing your posture and noticing how your behavior affects sensations in your neck and shoulders, can be extremely useful in finding lasting relief.

healing yoga practice to prevent & relieve neck & shoulder pain

One of the most important questions I ask new students is: "What do you hope to gain through the practice of yoga?" I ask this question for two reasons. One, it's useful for me to know what brings someone to yoga so that I have an understanding of their expectations and needs. Two, it's useful for students to clarify, in their own minds, what they want from yoga practice.

The yogic term for this process is *samkalpa*. Generally translated as "intention," samkalpa is a desire or wish that you clearly state or affirm, like a New Year's resolution, to help channel your energies to move in a particular direction. This concept recognizes the importance of the mind-body connection and highlights yoga's power to harness the mind for healing and spiritual development. If you aimlessly step onto your yoga mat and mindlessly move through the motions, the result is likely to be quite different, and less effective, than if you set an intention for your practice and then move diligently along your chosen path.

Judging from the replies I receive, two of the most common gains people hope to realize through yoga are flexibility and stress reduction. Other typical answers—such as relaxation, better sleep, and peace—are reflections of the nearly ubiquitous desire to ease stress. In fact, when I ask students for "special requests" at the beginning of class, someone often blurts out, only partly in jest, "Let's just do savasana (relaxation pose) today." Other students laugh, nodding in agreement, acknowledging their need to release stress and reconnect with the sense of peace and stillness cultivated in this final relaxation pose.

Yet as hungry as people are for stress relief, most find it surprisingly difficult to go straight from a busy day into stillness. Asked to sit or lie quietly, they begin fidgeting—tapping their fingers, wiggling their legs, or scrunching their faces—as their active minds continue to chatter and their tense bodies seek release. This is why yoga practice moves sequentially, beginning with *centering* to make the important transition from our typical focus outward, which emphasizes doing, to the sacred drawing inward of attention, which emphasizes simply *being*. *Breath awareness* is an important part of this shift, since our breath helps us connect the body and mind, and brings us into the present moment. Next come *postures* to release physical and mental tension; enhance energy flow; and cultivate strength, endurance, and flexibility. This, in turn, prepares us for *meditation*, where we come into stillness and connect with our true self.

The soft, peaceful expressions of people after yoga practice are often startlingly different from their rushed, tense faces before class. I've often been tempted to take "before" and "after" pictures of my students' faces to highlight this amazing transition from stressed and tight to relaxed and blissful. I'd entitle this photo gallery, "This Is Your Brain on Yoga."

practice overview

Since this book is devoted to healing neck and shoulder pain, this practice is designed to enhance flexibility and strength in these areas—and you'll see that an entire section is devoted to postures specific to the neck, shoulders, arms, upper back, and face. But as a holistic discipline, yoga recognizes that pain in one area of the body is likely to be related to imbalances elsewhere. So for true healing, it's also essential to cultivate strength, flexibility, and good alignment throughout the body to support and enhance neck and shoulder health, which is why this practice includes six parts:

1. *Centering and Breathing:* These awareness and breathing practices help you focus your mind, deepen your respiration, and connect your mind and body through your breath.

2. *Whole-Body Stretch:* This series of warm-up postures is designed to release tension, enhance circulation, and boost energy flow throughout your body.

3. *Standing Poses:* These poses enhance strength, balance, mobility, stability, and confidence. Learning to stand on our own two feet (and sometimes on one foot!) with good alignment is essential to our physical and psychological health.

4. *Neck and Shoulder Poses:* These postures are designed to release tension, enhance strength, and boost flexibility in this area, including the neck, shoulders, upper back, arms, hands, and face.

5. *Back-Bending Poses:* These dynamic and energizing poses help strengthen your back, enhancing back health and countering tendencies toward rounded shoulders and forward head posture.

6. *Deep Relaxation:* This yogic practice, called *savasana* or "corpse pose," is a head-to-toe tension reliever that teaches us the surprisingly difficult art of letting go and surrendering completely to the earth.

when to practice

Ideally, you'd do the entire practice every day, which will take about forty-five minutes to an hour. But if this is too great a time commitment, it's fine to do less. Even as little as five minutes of practice a day can offer significant benefit, according to the renowned Indian yoga master, T. K. V. Desikachar. I had an opportunity to interview Mr. Desikachar for a *Yoga Journal* article (Krucoff 2007), and he told me that he always asks new students how much time they have for daily practice. If someone tells him they only have five minutes, he designs a five-minute practice. He stressed that it's important to meet people where they are and find an amount of time they can commit to, rather than insist they practice for a longer period that they might find difficult or even skip entirely.

> *A short practice you do regularly is better than a long practice you rarely have time for.*

The bottom line is that a short practice you do regularly is better than a long practice you rarely have time for. In other words, it's better to do some yoga every day than a lot of yoga once in a while. Mr. Desikachar says (Krucoff 2007) that daily practice, even for a short time, helps create the yoga habit. He finds that people who start with five minutes a day typically feel so much better that they see the value and benefit of practice and then make time to do more.

It's most important to make a commitment to regular practice. So decide how long you can devote to your yoga practice and commit to doing some yoga every day. For example, if you only have fifteen minutes a day, you might (1) spend three minutes breathing and centering, (2) eight minutes doing the whole-body stretch (or standing poses or back-bending poses), and then (3) four minutes doing neck and shoulder poses. Be sure that, over a week's time, you've practiced most of the postures at least twice. And perhaps once a week, commit to a longer session, where you do the entire practice.

In our hyperbusy world, lack of time is often cited as the greatest barrier to personal practice. But when you recognize that the average American spends four hours a day watching TV, it becomes clear that, for many people, this perceived lack of time is an excuse. True reasons for not practicing often have more to do with other factors, such as exhaustion, fear, laziness, and guilt. How you spend your time is a matter of making choices, which means that you may need to give up something to gain the fifteen to sixty minutes a day you'll devote to yoga. Maybe this "sacrifice" will be giving up some time surfing the Internet, talking on the phone, watching TV, or shopping. The good news is that the time you spend doing yoga will be more than made up by the increased energy, flexibility, strength, balance, and calm the practice brings.

The best way to form the habit of practicing yoga is to schedule your session at the same time each day. Because postures should be practiced on an empty stomach, it's important to pick a time that's at least two hours after a major meal or an hour after a snack. This is one reason why early morning, before any food is eaten, is traditionally the time for yoga practice. In addition, early morning is thought to have energetic benefits. The ancient yogis considered the time just before sunrise (called *Brahma-muhurta*, or the hour of the god Brahma) to be the best time for practice, because the atmosphere is most highly charged with prana, which, as previously mentioned, is the Sanskrit word for vital energy or the life force. Modern research suggests that people who exercise first thing in the morning are more likely to stick with their programs. In our culture, few obligations compete with an early-morning practice time, and morning sessions are less likely to be skipped because of extra work or family duties that pop up unexpectedly. Another good time for practice is after work and before dinner. Your stomach is likely to be relatively empty, and the act of shedding work clothes and moving onto your mat can be a welcome opportunity to embrace the "undoing" quality of yoga. A predinner practice can be a great way to release the stress of the workday—a true "happy hour" for body and soul.

The best time for your practice is whatever works in your life!

Late evening may be suitable for a gentle, restorative practice or meditation. But it's inadvisable to do a vigorous practice or one that includes back bends (which are energizing) right before bed, because you may have difficulty falling asleep as a result. Depending on your schedule, late morning or before lunch may be a lovely time for a midday yoga break. The bottom line is that the best time for your practice is whatever works in your life!

And, paradoxically, as important as it is to make practice a part of your life, it's equally important to avoid being too rigid. One of the principles of the yogic path is nonattachment, even to the practice of *asanas* (yoga postures). This is one reason why, traditionally, no asana practice is done on new-moon and full-moon days. So on days when you're tired or not feeling well, either physically or emotionally, it's fine to set your timer for ten to fifteen (or more) minutes and just do centering and breathing, deep relaxation, or both. Because yoga is as much about undoing as doing, sometimes the most appropriate and healing practice will involve lying still and focusing on your breath. But yoga is also about balance, so, unless you're ill, it's important to practice the more active postures too.

And remember that yoga becomes most powerful when you don't confine your practice to the time you spend on the mat. As much as possible, weave postures from this series into your day, such as doing hug arms at your desk, shoulder shrugs while waiting on "hold" on the phone, or lion's face in the shower. Anytime you're standing in line—at the bank, in the grocery store, or at the post office, for example—practice mountain pose. (See chapter 6, "Off-the-Mat Practices.") These postures will help you bring your awareness to places where you habitually hold tension; learn to release chronic holding; and stretch and strengthen your muscles to support your head, shoulders, and neck with healthy alignment.

Whatever amount of time you take to practice, remember that it's better to do a few postures well than rush through a lot of postures poorly, because with yoga, it's not just *what* you do, but *how you do it*, that matters.

(Some of the material in this section was reprinted by permission of Powered, Inc., from the author's 2003 work, the "Yoga for Everyone" course for Powered, Inc., Austin, Texas.)

how to practice

If you're used to the Western approach to exercise, where the harder you work, the better the results, you may find yoga particularly challenging. But it's not that the postures are so difficult. What's so hard for many Americans is learning to embrace the "nonstriving" mind-set essential to yoga practice. For those of us steeped in cultural messages of "no pain, no gain," "go for the gold," and "give it your all," learning to adopt the yogic approach of balancing effort with surrender may take some getting used to.

In yoga, we recognize that working hard may actually create *more* tension and take you farther away from where you want to be. So, rather than "muscling into" a pose, which can lead to injury, we learn that relaxing into a pose can actually take us deeper. Yoga teaches us to become keenly aware of how the pose feels, take the movement to a point of challenge but not strain, and allow the breath to invite the posture to unfold.

In other words, we typically progress in yoga not by working harder, but by working *softer*—relaxing, releasing, and letting go; or better yet, by not *working* at the pose at all, but by *playing* with it, which means:

- Starting where we are (not where we think we should be).

- Accepting and loving ourselves just as we are.

- Being honest about how the pose feels (and if it hurts, backing off!).

- Letting go of our ego and concerns about how we look or how we compare to others.

- Being present with our breath and staying present in our bodies (not thinking about work, other people, or what's on TV).

- Taking each pose to a point of mild tension but *never* to pain.

- Being patient; just as you can't force a rosebud to open, time and practice are essential to making progress.

- Having fun. Remember that feeling as a child, when the recess bell rang and released you out onto the playground to run, jump, and swing and do whatever your little heart and body desired? Yoga offers that opportunity for a daily recess. So recognize that your practice is not just about building strength and flexibility; it's also a precious opportunity to enjoy the sensations of moving your body through space, to breathe deeply and feel your limbs surge with energy. It's a chance to express gratitude for the gift of your body and your breath.

practice principles

As you practice, please remember these yogic ABCs:

Awareness: See if, during your entire practice, you can keep your mind present in your body, focused on your breath and your experience in the present moment. If your mind spins off toward anything but your breath and your pose, please notice without judgment that your mind is chattering, and release those thoughts like a child letting go of a helium balloon, allowing the distractions to float away. Then bring your attention back to your breath and your pose.

Breathing: Keep your breathing slow, deep, and even as you practice. If you find that you can't breathe slowly and deeply, it's a sign that you're straining, so back off the postures and come to a place where you can breathe slowly and deeply. In this way, our breath becomes our teacher, letting us know if we're under stress.

Balance: Approach your practice with a balance of doing and undoing, effort and surrender, courage and caution. Don't be lazy, but don't be pushy either!

Comfort and Stability: The ancient texts on yoga tell us that a posture should be "steady and comfortable" or, according to some translations, "relaxed and stable" or "sweet and calm." So if you're straining to achieve a posture suitable for a calendar photo, that's gymnastics or calisthenics but not yoga. The yogic approach is to move into each posture only to the point where you feel a sensation of pleasant stretch, then allow your breath to help the pose deepen and unfold.

It's also critical to understand that, like any form of physical activity, yoga carries the risk of injury. Typically, when people get injured doing yoga, it's because they're overzealous and pushing themselves in their practice, in other words, ignoring all those principles previously listed about nonstriving and never straining, pushing, or forcing. And it's also important to recognize that not every posture is appropriate for every person. While the poses in the sequence offered in this chapter are generally safe for most people, if you have health concerns or are taking medications for a chronic condition, it's always advisable to check with your health care provider before beginning yoga or any new form of physical activity.

Remember that yoga should never be painful. If any of these postures hurts or doesn't feel right, please don't do it! (If you have serious health issues, consider consulting an experienced yoga teacher or yoga therapist for individualized instruction; to find one in your area, see the resources section.)

where to practice

You don't need a separate room for your practice, but it can be helpful to create a "sacred space" in a corner or section of a room that has a nonslip, level surface, such as a hardwood floor or a firm rug. A yoga "sticky mat" can be very helpful (see the resources section), but it's also fine to use a beach towel or blanket to practice the reclining poses, and a firm surface to practice the standing poses.

It's most important to eliminate distractions. If you can, practice behind a closed door in a quiet room. Be sure to turn off the ringer on your home and cell phones, allowing any messages to go to voice mail. Ask others to respect your need for concentration during practice and to avoid interrupting you. Some people enjoy using meditative background music to help set a peaceful tone; others prefer silence.

You might consider decorating your practice area with an inspiring picture or pleasing piece of artwork to enhance the meditative quality of the space. A timer can be useful if you have only a specific amount of time for your practice. This way, you can set the timer to ring when you need to wrap up, eliminating the distracting need to check the clock.

The Practice

centering and breathing

1. **Centering:** Lie on your back with your knees bent, your feet flat on the floor, and your arms resting at your sides. Relax your shoulders and your neck. (If your chin "pokes up," place a folded towel or blanket under your head so that if you were viewed from the side, your forehead and chin would be level. Be sure your neck retains its natural curve; don't flatten your neck by elevating your head too high.) Soften your face and release the hinge of your jaw so that your teeth gently part and the inside of your mouth softens. If you're comfortable closing your eyes, do so. But if you'd prefer to leave your eyes open, that's fine; just keep your gaze soft, looking at nothing in particular. Bring your attention to your breath.

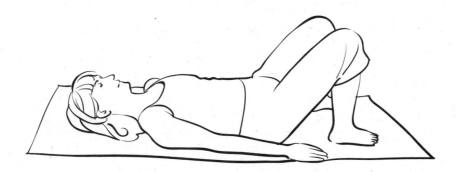

Figure 5.1. Centering, Breath Awareness,
Body Scan, and Exhaling Tension

2. **Breath Awareness:** Watch the movement of breath in and out of your body and observe all the sensations associated with your breathing. Perhaps you'll notice the coolness of the air as it enters your nostrils and feel the warmth as it exits. You might feel your torso expanding on inhalation and contracting on exhalation. Notice the quality and the texture of your breath in this moment; is it deep and slow, or perhaps short and choppy? Follow your inhalation all the way to the end and notice the little pause at the end of your inbreath as it makes the transition to an outbreath. Then follow your exhalation all the way to the end, and notice that there's another brief pause as the outbreath makes the shift to become an inbreath. As best you can, stay with your breath, observing, without judgment, where the breath goes and where it doesn't go.

3. **Body Scan:** Check in with yourself and see what's going on for you today; notice how you feel physically and also how you feel mentally and emotionally. With your mind's eye, take an inward journey through your body and mind, scanning your whole interior landscape, looking for any places of tension or tightness, any discomfort or "dis-ease," any pain or holding. And if you find places like this, send your breath there, inviting softness and release.

4. **Exhaling Tension:** Bring your attention to the back of your body and notice all the places where you're touching the earth, such as your back and buttocks, the back of your head, the backs of your arms, and the soles of your feet. Feel this connection with the floor that supports you. Recognize that the floor will hold you up without any effort on your part. See if, with each exhalation, you can let go just a little more into the support of the floor underneath you. With each exhalation, allow your body to become heavier and more relaxed, releasing more and more of its weight into the earth. Let each inhalation be an opportunity to fill your body with breath, and allow each exhalation to be a chance to relax and let go of anything you don't need, surrendering more and more of your body weight into the earth.

5. **Deep Abdominal Breath:** Place your hands on your lower belly, resting your palms above your pubic bone but below your navel. On your next inhalation, invite the air all the way down to the lowest portion of your lungs, and notice how, when you fill your lungs completely this way, your belly rounds and your hands gently rise. Then observe how, as you exhale and let all the air out of your lungs, your belly releases down and your hands gently fall. Continue for a few more slow, deep breaths, watching this gentle rise and fall: take an easy, full breath in so that the belly rounds and the hands gently rise; and release an easy, full breath out so that the belly relaxes down and the hands gently fall.

Now, as you continue to breathe slowly and deeply, visualize your lungs as two big balloons that extend all the way down to your belly, into your side ribs and up under your collarbones. On your inhalation, imagine these balloons expanding completely in six directions: side to side, top to bottom, and front to back. Notice how the belly rounds and also how your rib cage swells out to the sides like an accordion filling with air. On your exhalation, release all the old, used air, gently engaging your abdominal muscles at the end of the exhalation so that your belly hugs in toward your spine and squeezes out the old, used breath. Then relax your belly completely so that it's soft and receptive as you fill your lungs once again with fresh, new breath.

On each inhalation, the belly rounds, the rib cage expands out to the sides, and the upper chest fills and broadens. On each exhalation, everything softens and the belly hugs toward the spine, pressing out the old, stale air. Continue this deep, full breathing for five to six complete rounds of breath.

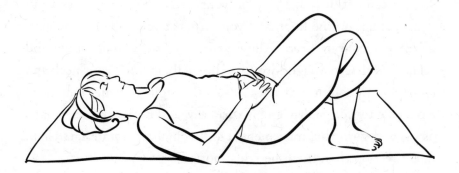

Figure 5.2. Deep Abdominal Breath

whole-body stretch

6.　**Neck Release:** Lying on your back with your knees bent, your feet flat on the floor, and your arms at your sides, bring your awareness to your head. Allow your head to become heavy and relaxed so that its weight drops to the earth, inviting your neck and shoulders to soften and release. Gently begin rocking your head from side to side, slowly and luxuriously, and notice the sensations associated with this movement. Does your head rotate farther in one direction than the other? Just notice.

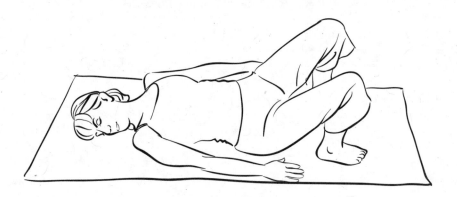

Figure 5.3. Neck Release

7. **Neck Stretch:** Center your head by lining your chin up with the little notch in the middle of your collarbones. Take a big breath in, and on the exhalation, turn your head to the right as far as it will comfortably go so that your chin moves in the direction of your right shoulder. Rest here for a few breaths. Drop your left shoulder down toward the floor and send your breath into the left side of your neck, inviting softness and release. On an inhalation, bring your head back to center and then exhale your head to the left as far as it will comfortably go, moving your chin in the direction of your left shoulder and resting there for a few breaths. Drop your right shoulder down into the floor and send your breath into the right side of your neck, inviting softness and release. When you're ready, inhale back to the center.

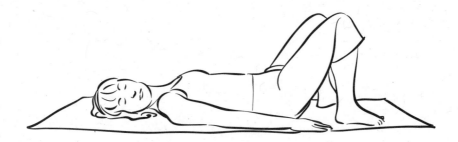

Figure 5.4. Neck Stretch

8. **Upper Back and Shoulder Stretch:** Rest your arms by your sides and tune in to your breath. On an inhalation, extend your arms up and overhead so that the backs of your hands come to the floor behind you, or as close to the floor as they will comfortably go. Then on an exhalation, stretch your arms back up and bring them back down beside you. Continue with this simple movement—inhaling up and back, exhaling forward and down—for eight to ten slow, deep breaths. Synchronize your movement with your breath and bend your elbows as much as you need to for comfort. Move slowly and with intention, as if you're moving through water. Don't rush to get your hands to the floor; keep everything moving and fluid, enjoying your breath.

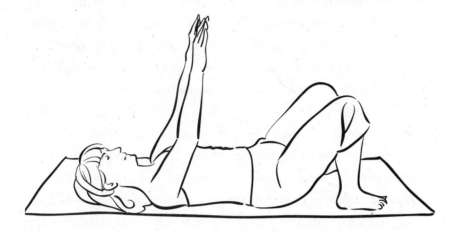

Figure 5.5a. Upper Back and Shoulder Stretch: Arms to the Sky

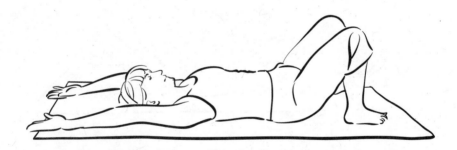

Figure 5.5b. Upper Back and Shoulder Stretch: Arms Overhead

9. **Single-Knee-to-Chest Pose with Ankle Circles:** Lying with your knees bent, your feet on the floor, and arms at your sides, take a nice deep breath in. On an exhalation, hug your right knee into your chest, holding your leg behind your right thigh. (If this is a strain on your shoulders, please use a yoga strap, or an old necktie or bathrobe belt, to catch your leg.) Stay here for a few breaths, drawing your right thigh in toward your rib cage each time you exhale and noticing the sensation of stretching. Continuing to hug your leg, imagine that your big toe is a crayon and begin slowly drawing large circles in the air to wake up the ankles. Then reverse the direction and draw a few more slow, easy circles in the opposite direction.

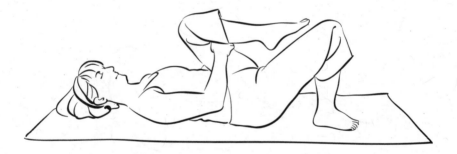

Figure 5.6. Single-Knee-to-Chest Pose

10. **Leg Stretch:** Continue to hug your right leg and, on an inhalation, extend your right foot up toward the sky, straightening your leg as much as you comfortably can. Then exhale and bend your knee so that your foot comes back down by your buttocks. On your next inhalation, straighten your leg back up, with your foot extending up toward the sky, and repeat this movement— exhale and bend, inhale and straighten—three to five times, moving with the breath. Then relax and repeat postures 9 and 10 with the left leg.

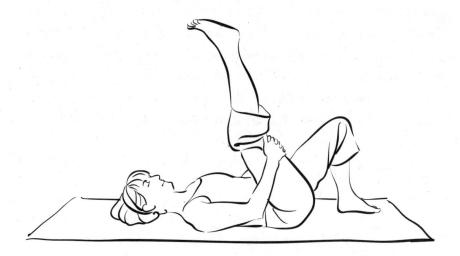

Figure 5.7. Leg Stretch

11. **Both-Knees-to-Chest Pose:** With both feet on the ground and both knees bent, take a deep, full breath in. On an exhalation, hug both knees in toward your chest, holding behind your thighs or above your shins with your hands, or catching the legs with a strap if that's more comfortable. Bring your awareness to the sensations of stretching in your lower back and buttocks. On the inhalation, feel your lungs fill completely with breath and expand so that your arms straighten and your thighs gently float away from your belly. On the exhalation, hug your belly toward your spine as you bend your elbows and draw your thighs even closer to your rib cage, stretching out your lower back. Repeat five to ten times, moving with the breath: inhale and expand, letting your thighs float away; exhale and draw in, belly to spine and thighs toward chest. Notice the gentle pumping action that's so helpful to the digestion. When you've finished, release your legs so that your feet come back to the floor, roll over onto your side, and use the strength of your hands and arms to come up onto all fours.

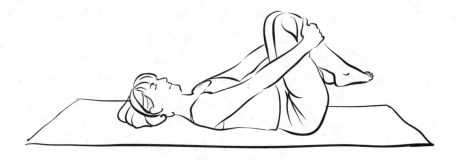

Figure 5.8a. Both-Knees-to-Chest Pose: Legs Away

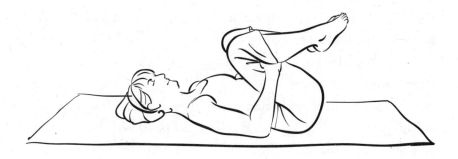

Figure 5.8b. Both-Knees-to-Chest Pose: Legs In

12. **Cat Pose and Dog Tilt:** Bring your hands directly under your shoulders and your knees directly under your hips. Be sure your knees are comfortable; you may want to place a folded towel or blanket under them for extra padding. Fan your fingers out wide along the floor, pressing evenly into the floor with the pads and base of each finger. If you have any wrist discomfort, support them with a folded towel, or come up onto your fists. From this position, called "table pose," inhale fully and completely, lengthening the spine so that the crown of your head reaches forward and your tailbone reaches back. On an exhalation, arch your spine up into a dome like an angry Halloween cat, as you release your tailbone and your head down toward the floor into "cat pose." On an inhalation, release your spine down toward the ground so that it curves in the opposite direction, like a hammock, and your collarbones and head lift gently, keeping your neck long, and your tailbone rises. This is "dog tilt." Soften your face and let your gaze rise up toward the sky.

Continue alternating these movements with your breath—exhaling and arching your back up into cat pose, and then inhaling and releasing your spine down into dog tilt. Keep the movement slow and mindful, and tune in to the sensations of flexing and extending your spine. See if you can feel each individual vertebra moving one by one, like a string of pearls, as you arch your back up into cat pose on exhalation and release your back down to dog tilt on inhalation. Be sure to let your head drop down completely in cat pose to release the muscles in your neck. Repeat five to ten times, moving with the breath.

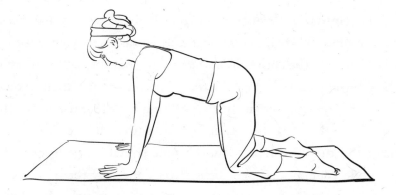

Figure 5.9a. Cat Pose and Dog Tilt: Table Pose

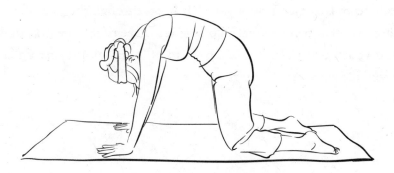

Figure 5.9b. Cat Pose and Dog Tilt: Cat Pose

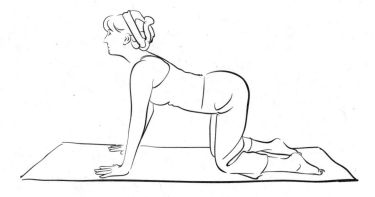

Figure 5.9c. Cat Pose and Dog Tilt: Dog Tilt

13. **Spinal Balance:** Begin on all fours, with a flat back, in table pose. Take a nice, deep breath in and feel your rib cage expand around the entire circumference of your torso. On an exhalation, bring your right knee forward, and on an inhalation, extend your right leg back so that the toes of your right foot reach straight behind you. Do this three times to build up heat in the body. At the end of the third repetition, continue stretching your leg back, extending your toes straight behind you, and stay there for a few breaths. If you want an extra challenge, pick up your left hand and extend your left arm forward, reaching through your fingertips and feeling the long, diagonal line of energy extending through your body from the fingertips of your left hand through the toes of your right foot. Keep your breath flowing for three to five breaths; don't hold your breath. Then come back to all fours and repeat on the other side.

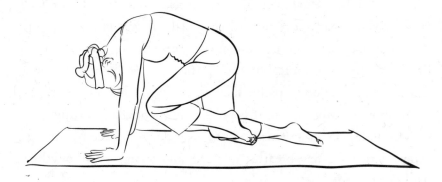

Figure 5.10a. Spinal Balance: Prep

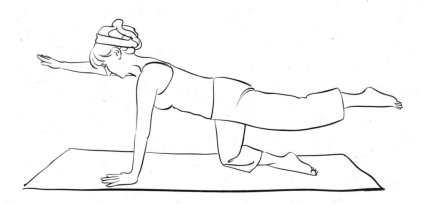

· Figure 5.10b. Spinal Balance: Challenge

14. **Child's Pose:** Bring your buttocks back toward your heels and let your head move toward the earth. If you like, stack your palms or fists on the floor and rest your forehead on your hands, or if your forehead comfortably reaches the floor, rest your arms along the sides of your body, palms facing up. If you have a round body, to be more comfortable in this pose, you might try spreading your thighs wide, allowing your body to ease down between your legs. Stay there for a few breaths, relaxing and letting go of anything you don't need.

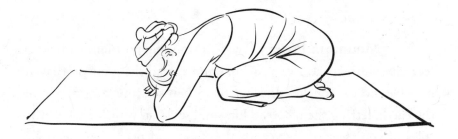

Figure 5.11a. Child's Pose

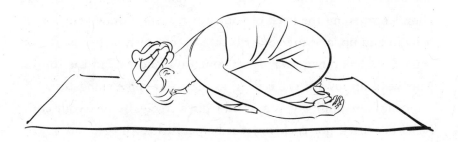

Figure 5.11b. Child's Pose: Arms at Sides

standing poses for strength and balance

15. **Mountain Pose:** Come to a standing position, with your feet hip-width apart. Lift your toes and spread them out so that, if possible, no toe touches another toe. Then set your toes down on the earth, letting them spread long and wide on your mat. Feel the soles of your feet connect with the floor, and press down equally with all four "corners" of your feet—the base of the big toe, the base of the little toe, the inner heel, and the outer heel—so that you feel grounded and stable. From this place of grounding, invite the energy to rise up your legs, as if you were a tree drawing up nutrients from the earth. Release your tailbone down toward the floor, lengthening the back of your waist. Gently draw your lower belly in and up, and lift your rib cage up out of your pelvis. Relax your shoulders down away from your ears, and extend the top of your head up toward the ceiling so that your spine elongates as if someone were pulling you upward from a string. Be sure your chin is neither lifted nor tucked; let it be parallel to the ground. Gaze softly toward the horizon, with your shoulders, throat, and face relaxed. Imagine a light shining out from your heart center, right at your breastbone, and be sure it shines forward, not down at the ground. Take several slow, full breaths, filling and emptying your lungs completely and imagining yourself as strong and stable as a mountain.

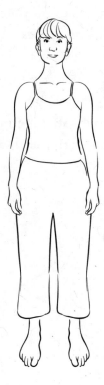

Figure 5.12. Mountain Pose

16. **Standing Salutation:** Standing in mountain pose, turn your palms out, and on an inhalation, extend your arms out to the sides and up overhead until your palms touch, lifting your heart toward the sky and gazing up at your thumbs. Be sure to keep your neck long; don't drop your head back. As you exhale, keep your palms together and bring your hands down past your forehead and throat, and let them rest in prayer position at your heart. Repeat five times, synchronizing your movement with your breath. On the inhalation visualize yourself gathering in positive energy; on the exhalation bring this energy into your heart.

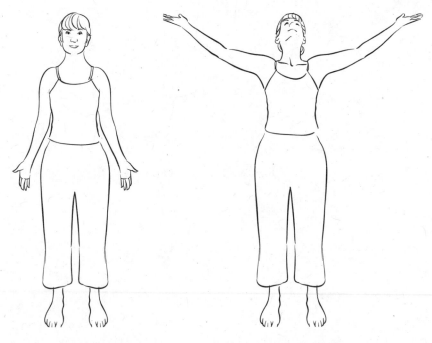

Figure 5.13a. Standing
Salutation: Arms Down

Figure 5.13b. Standing
Salutation: Arms Up and Out

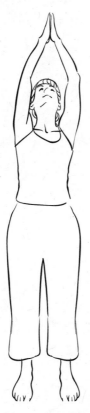

Figure 5.13c. Standing Salutation: Arms Up and Palms Together

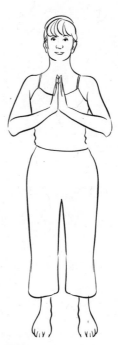

Figure 5.13d. Standing Salutation: Arms in Prayer Position

17. **Mountain Pose Variation—Arm Up/Head Turn:**
Standing in mountain pose, take a deep breath and exhale completely. On your next inhalation, extend your right arm forward and up, and turn your head to the left, keeping your shoulders squared off toward the front so that only your neck and head turn. On the exhalation, return your head to center and relax your arm down by your side. On the next inhalation, inhale your left arm up and turn your head to the right, and then exhale back to the starting position. As best you can, try to keep your shoulders relaxed down away from your ears when you lift your arm up. Repeat five times, alternating sides and synchronizing your movement with your breath.

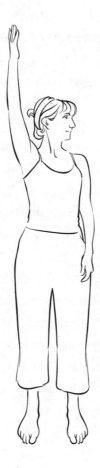

Figure 5.14. Mountain Pose Variation—Arm Up/Head Turn

18. **Tree Pose:** Begin in mountain pose, feeling your body weight evenly distributed on both legs and the crown of your head extending up toward the sky. (If you want some extra support, practice this balancing posture near a wall or sturdy chair that you can touch lightly if needed.) On an inhalation, extend your arms out to the sides, at about shoulder height, reaching the fingers of your right hand out to the right and the fingers of your left hand out to the left. Exhale and relax your shoulders down away from your ears. Then keep your breath flowing easily in and out as you imagine sending roots down through your right leg and foot into the ground. Pick up your left heel, keeping the ball of your left foot on the floor. Turn your left knee out slightly to the left as you slide the sole of your left foot against your right ankle. This may be your tree pose, and if so, that's wonderful. Just stay there and breathe.

If you'd like more of a challenge, pick your left foot up off the floor and place the sole anywhere you'd like along the inside of your right leg. But avoid pressing your foot directly against your knee; pick a spot either above or below the knee. Bring your hands together at your heart center, in prayer position. For more of a challenge, extend your arms up overhead, making sure to keep your shoulders relaxed and down, away from your ears. Gaze softly at a fixed spot on the horizon; this point of focus is called your *drishti*, and anchoring your gaze here aids concentration and can help stabilize your balance. Extend up through the crown of your

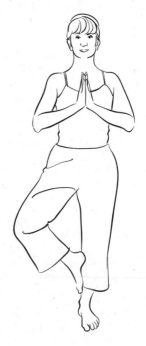

Figure 5.15a. Tree Pose

head as you root down through your right leg and foot. Feel free to touch your toe back to the earth anytime you need to, or touch the wall or a chair for support. If you lose your balance, take a breath and try again. Stay here for five slow, deep breaths, and then bring your foot down and repeat on the other side.

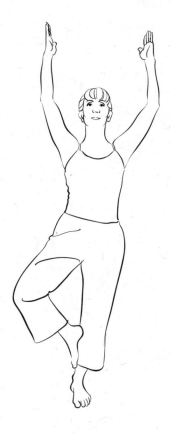

**Figure 5.15b. Tree Pose:
Arms Up**

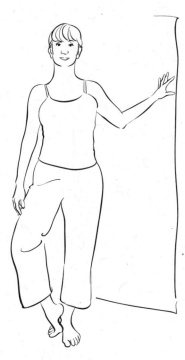

**Figure 5.15c. Tree Pose
Modified: Toe Touch**

19. **Puppy Dog:** Practice this pose next to a wall, chair, or countertop, such as a desk or kitchen counter. Place your palms on the chair back, wall, or countertop, and walk your feet back until your arms are fully extended in front of you. Then hinge forward at the hips, and continue walking back until your torso is parallel to the floor and your hips are directly over your ankles. Bring your feet shoulder-width apart, and press your palms into the countertop or wall as your draw your hips back and straighten your legs as best you can. Stay there for several slow, deep breaths, feeling the stretch in your back and along the backs of your legs. Keep your hands pressing into the solid surface and your hips extending back. Then, as you're ready, walk your feet forward and release.

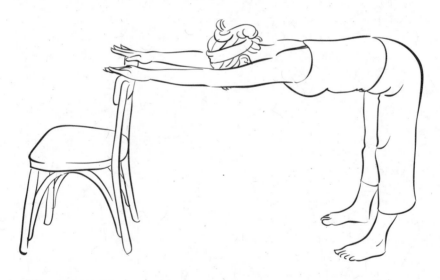

Figure 5.16. Puppy Dog

20. **Gentle Twist:** Standing in mountain pose, with the crown of your head extending up toward the sky and your feet planted firmly on the ground, turn your body gently to the right so that, if possible, you can see behind you over your right shoulder. Then come back through the center, and turn your body gently to the left so that, if possible, you can see behind you over your left shoulder. Continue this gentle turning to both sides, allowing your arms to be soft and "noodly" by your sides for three to five slow, easy breaths.

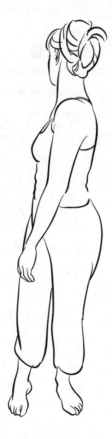

Figure 5.17. Gentle Twist

poses to stretch and strengthen the neck and shoulders

The postures in this section are shown seated on a chair, rather than seated on the floor, for several reasons. First, I'd like to encourage you to practice them throughout your day, for example, while you're at your desk. Second, sitting cross-legged on the floor with good posture is extremely difficult, and sometimes impossible, for many people in Western cultures. If you'd like, you can also do most of these postures while standing in mountain pose (posture 15).

21. **Seated Mountain Pose:** Sit tall in your chair, with your feet planted firmly on the ground and your sit bones (see chapter 4, "Sitting Pretty") dropping down into the seat of the chair. From this place of grounding, extend the crown of your head up toward the sky, lengthening your spine. Relax your shoulders down away from your ears and let your hands rest on your thighs. Be sure your chin is parallel to the ground, neither poking up nor tucked in. Imagine that you have a headlight in the center of your chest at your breastbone, and shine that light forward (not down toward the ground). Relax your face. With a soft gaze and smiling eyes, look toward the horizon.

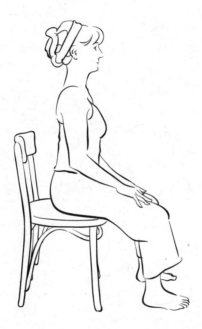

Figure 5.18. Seated Mountain Pose

22. **Shoulder Shrugs:** Inhale your shoulders up toward your ears, and then exhale and drop them down. Inhale and squeeze them up; exhale and release them down. Repeat several times, making sure to keep your arms as relaxed as possible so that they go along for the ride. For an extra challenge and to build strength in the upper back, try this raised-arm version: Inhale your arms up overhead, palms facing each other. From this position, inhale your shoulders up toward your ears; then exhale and drop them down. Repeat three to five times, synchronizing your movement with your breath.

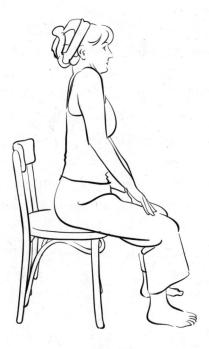

Figure 5.19. Shoulder Shrug

23. **Shoulder Clock:** Lift your shoulders up as high as they'll comfortably go—we'll call this "twelve o'clock,"—take them back to "nine o'clock," release them down to "six o'clock," and then bring them forward to "three o'clock." Keep your breath slow and deep as you continue circling your shoulders around the entire face of this imaginary clock several times; then reverse direction, taking the shoulders up, then forward, then down, then back. Let the movement be easy and "juicy," getting as much motion as possible in your shoulders. For an extra challenge, try bicycling your shoulders so that the right shoulder goes up while the left shoulder goes down, the right shoulder goes forward while the left shoulder goes back, the right shoulder goes down while the left shoulder goes up, and the right shoulder goes back while the left shoulder goes forward; then reverse direction.

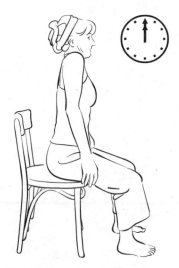

Figure 5.20a. Shoulder Clock:
Twelve o'Clock

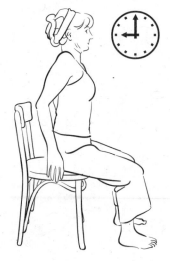

Figure 5.20b. Shoulder Clock:
Nine o'Clock

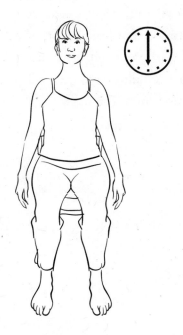

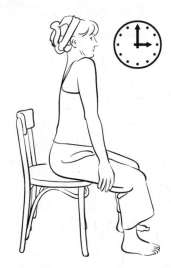

Figure 5.20c. Shoulder Clock:
Six o'Clock

Figure 5.20d. Shoulder Clock:
Three o'Clock

24. **Hug Arms:** On an inhalation, extend your arms out to the sides at shoulder height; on an exhalation, relax your shoulders down away from your ears, continuing to reach your arms out so that the fingers of your right hand extend to the right and the fingers of your left hand extend to the left. Inhale your "wingspan" out as wide as you can; then exhale and hug yourself, feeling your shoulder blades move away from each other in your back. Inhale as you lengthen the crown of your head toward the sky; then exhale as you drop your chin to your chest and lift your chest to your chin. Notice which arm you chose to put on top. Stay there for several breaths, stretching out the back of your neck and your upper back; then inhale your head back up and extend your arms back out to the sides. Repeat, this time placing the other arm on top in the hug.

Try this hug arms variation: Inhale your arms out to the sides; then exhale and hug with your right arm on top. Inhale your arms out to the sides; then exhale and hug with your left arm on top. Continue for five to ten breaths, synchronizing your movement with your breath and alternating the top arm in the hug.

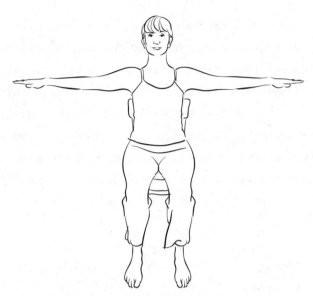

Figure 5.21a. Hug Arms: Arms Extended

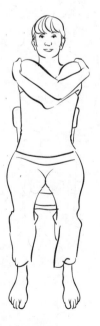

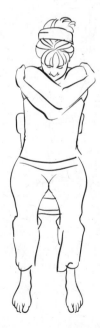

Figure 5.21b. Hug Arms:
Head Level

Figure 5.21c. Hug Arms:
Head Down

25. **Angel Wings:** Extend your arms forward; then bend your elbows and place your fingertips on your shoulders. On an inhalation, open your elbows out to the sides and draw your shoulder blades together in the back of your body, as if you had a nut on your spine and your shoulder blades were moving together like a nutcracker squeezing the nut. On an exhalation, bring your elbows forward and together (or as close as they'll comfortably come) in front of you, and feel your shoulder blades sliding apart in back of your body. Continue for three to six breaths.

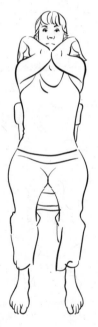

Figure 5.22a. Angel Wings: Forward

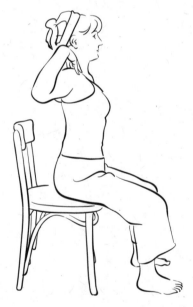

Figure 5.22b. Angel Wings: Back

26. **Angel-Wing Circles:** With your fingers resting lightly on your shoulders, imagine that your elbows are felt-tipped markers, and draw large ovals in the air with them. Keep the breath slow and easy as you circle in one direction for three to five breaths and then reverse direction for three to five more breaths.

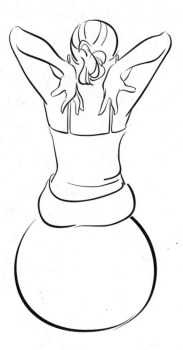

Figure 5.23. Angel-Wing Circles

27. **Seated Back Bend:** Sitting tall in seated mountain pose (posture 21), place your palms on your thighs and tuck your elbows in toward your sides. Imagine that you have a headlight shining out from the center of your chest at your breastbone. On an inhalation, lengthen the crown of your head toward the sky, and on an exhalation, press your palms into your thighs and your sit bones into the chair as you arch your back and lift your "headlight" so that it shines up toward the sky. Be sure to keep your neck long (don't drop your head back) and gaze up. Inhale back to the starting position. Repeat three to five times, moving with the breath; then relax.

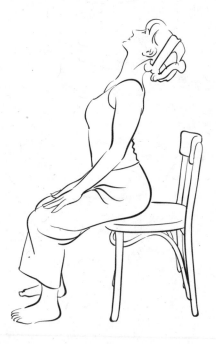

Figure 5.24. Seated Back Bend

28.

Head Turn: Inhale and lengthen the crown of your head toward the sky; exhale and turn your head as far to the right as possible, keeping your shoulders squared forward. Be sure to allow your eyes to be part of this turn, looking out the corners of your eyes toward whatever is behind you. Inhale back to the center; then exhale to the left. Repeat three to six times, moving with the breath.

To engage some of the deep muscles of your neck, try this pose with the fingers of your right hand lightly touching your right temple before you turn to the right, and see if you can initiate the head turn from this place at your temple, where you feel the gentle resistance of your fingers. Then repeat to the left.

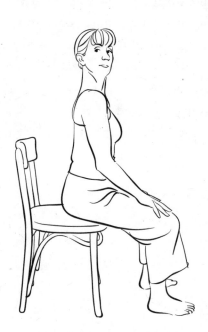

Figure 5.25a. Head Turn:
Eyes Leading

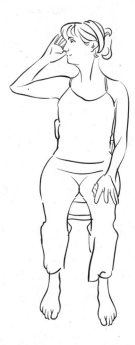

Figure 5.25b. Head Turn:
Fingers at Temple

29. **Ear to Shoulder:** Sitting tall in seated mountain pose, with your hands on your thighs, inhale as you lengthen the crown of your head toward the sky; then exhale and release your right ear down toward your right shoulder, trying not to lift the shoulder toward the ear. Drop your left shoulder down and breathe into the left side of your neck. Keep your breath flowing as you take your left hand off your thigh and let your left arm dangle down at your side. If you'd like, gently swing your arm like a pendulum, inviting the left arm, shoulder, and side of the neck to relax and release. Stay there for a few breaths, relaxing and letting go as best you can. Repeat on the other side.

For an extra challenge, from the right ear-to-shoulder position, sweep your left hand behind you and hold your right arm just above the elbow. Then exhale and gently rotate your head so that your nose moves toward your right shoulder. Inhale and rotate your head the other way so that your nose moves toward the sky. Continue for a few breaths, synchronizing your movement with your breath. Then relax, release your arms, and let your head float back over the shoulder girdle and the crown of the head, lifting to the sky. Repeat on the other side.

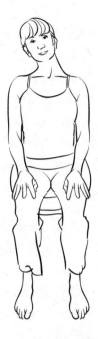

Figure 5.26a. Ear to Shoulder:
Hands on Thighs

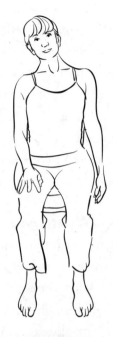

Figure 5.26b. Ear to Shoulder:
Arm Dangling

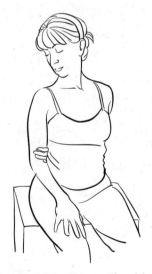

Figure 5.26c. Ear to Shoulder
Challenge: Down

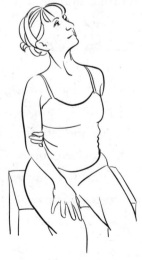

Figure 5.26d. Ear to Shoulder
Challenge: Up

30. **Bobblehead:** Sitting tall in mountain pose, imagine that you're a bobblehead doll, where the body is stable and the head bobbles around on a spring atop the neck. Keeping your spine long, begin to bobble your head gently, relaxing any tension in your neck and shoulders, for several breaths. Then bring your head into alignment over your shoulder girdle, as if it were a flower balanced on the stem of your neck, and come into stillness. Rest there for a few breaths.

31. **Wrist, Arm, and Side Stretch:** Clasp your hands together and inhale; then on an exhalation, extend your arms up and turn your palms away from you. (If this is not comfortable, do this with your palms facing toward you.) On an inhalation, lengthen through the crown of your head and extend your palms toward the sky, keeping your shoulders relaxed and down, away from your ears. On an exhalation, press down through your right sit bone and lean your upper body to the left. Inhale back to center; then exhale and press down through your left sit bone as you lean your upper body to the right. Continue three to five times, moving with the breath; then relax, bring your hands down into your lap, and switch the clasp of your hands. This means that, if you first clasped your hands with the right thumb on top of the left thumb and right index finger on top of the left index finger, now clasp them with the left thumb and index finger on top. Many people find this unaccustomed clasp surprisingly difficult, but that's part of the point: to bring your awareness to habitual patterns that you were previously unaware of and balance out your body. Once you've switched your clasp, repeat the stretch.

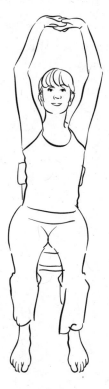
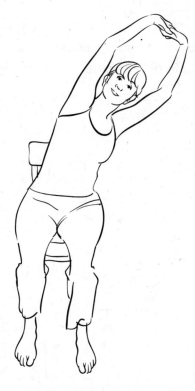

Figure 5.27a. Wrist, Arm, and Side Stretch

Figure 5.27b. Wrist, Arm, and Side Stretch

32. **Cow's-Face Arms:** Hold a yoga strap (or an old necktie or bathrobe belt) in your right hand and extend your right arm up overhead. Bend your right elbow so that it points up toward the sky and your right palm faces your upper back, with the strap resting along your back. Bend your left elbow and slide the back of your left hand up your back to hold the strap. Lengthen up through the crown of your head and relax your tailbone down toward the earth as you "walk" your hands toward each other along the strap. (If you can catch your hands without the strap—and without straining!—great. If not, great, too; use the strap.) Stop when you reach a point of pleasant stretch; then stay there for three to five slow, deep breaths. Relax and repeat on the other side.

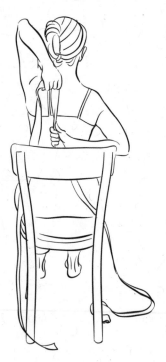

Figure 5.28. Cow's-Face Arms

33. **Lion's Face:** Take a deep, full breath in; then on an exhalation, open your mouth as wide as it will comfortably go, extending your tongue out as far as possible and opening your eyes as wide as you comfortably can while flinging your fingers out in front of you. As you do this, make a "haaaaa" sound with your exhalation and draw your belly in toward your spine. When you've exhaled completely, relax and take a few easy breaths. Repeat three to five times.

For an extra challenge, try extending your tongue toward your chin or toward your nose, and gaze in toward your nose. If you'd like (and you've notified anyone within hearing range that you're okay), roar loudly on exhalation.

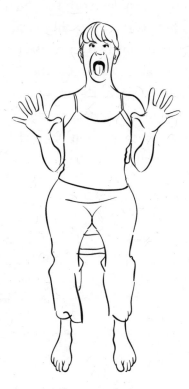

Figure 5.29. Lion's Face

poses to strengthen and stretch the back

34. **Crocodile Pose:** Come onto your belly on the floor, bend your elbows, and stack your hands to make a little pillow for your head, turning your neck so that your cheek or your ear rests on the back of your hands. If it's uncomfortable to turn your head in this position, please rest your forehead or chin on the backs of your hands. Allow your body to relax completely so that your weight releases down into the earth. If you'd like, let your heels drop out toward the outside edges of your mat, and angle your toes in toward each other. Take a few slow, deep breaths here and invite the back of your body to expand with the inhalation and relax on the exhalation. If you've turned your head, notice which side you turned it to; then switch, slowly turning your head the other way and resting the other ear or cheek on the backs of your hands. Notice how that feels. Observe the movement of your breath in the back portion of your lungs, feeling the back ribs expand on inhalation and release on exhalation. Completely surrender your body weight into the earth.

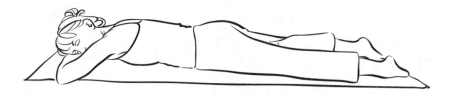

Figure 5.30. Crocodile Pose

35. **Modified Locust Pose:** Lying on your belly with your elbows bent and your hands stacked, place your forehead or your chin on the backs of your hands, whichever feels better to you. Bring your legs together and press the tops of your feet into the earth. Root down with your thighs, and drop your pubic bone down into the mat. On an inhalation, lift your right leg up, keeping it as straight as you comfortably can and reaching back with your toes. On an exhalation, return your leg to the earth. On your next inhalation, lift up your left leg, keeping it as straight as you comfortably can and reaching back with your toes. Then exhale it back down. Continue in this way for eight to twelve breaths, alternating legs, inhaling up, and exhaling down. Synchronize your movement with your breath and move as slowly as you comfortably can, staying present in your body and keeping your attention on the breath and the pose. If you need more of a challenge, keep your leg in the up position through several breath cycles. Be sure to keep breathing; don't hold your breath.

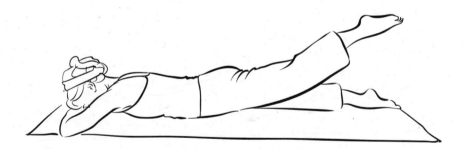

Figure 5.31. Modified Locust Pose

36.   **Baby Cobra:** Lying on your belly, bring your arms down by your sides and your chin or your forehead to the floor, placing a small folded towel under your forehead if you'd like. Root down through your pubic bone, and press your legs and the tops of your feet down into the earth, lengthening back through your feet. Find your breath. On an inhalation, lift your head, neck, shoulders, and upper back up as high as you comfortably can. On an exhalation, take everything back down. You may not be able to go up very high, and that's fine; just do the best you can. This is very strengthening for the upper back, and over time and with practice, you'll get stronger. Continue with this practice, inhaling up and exhaling down for three to six breaths. Be sure to keep your neck long so that you don't just crank your neck up and down but use your back muscles to lift the back and shoulders. To help lengthen the neck, imagine that you have an eye in the back of your neck, and try to keep that imaginary eye open. If you want more of a challenge, stay in the up position for several slow, deep breaths.

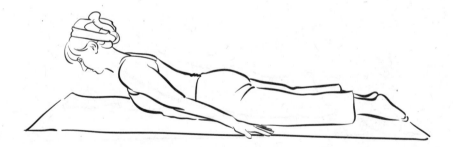

Figure 5.32. Baby Cobra

When you're finished, rest in crocodile pose (posture 34). Then take a moment to stretch out your back by placing your palms under your shoulders and pressing back to child's pose (posture 14). Relax there for a few breaths, inviting your lower back to soften and release.

37. **Bridge Pose:** Lie on your back with your knees bent and your feet hip-width apart, with your ankles under your knees. Rest your arms on the floor alongside your body with palms facing down and tune in to your breath. Take a nice, deep breath in; then, on an exhalation, press down with your feet and arms as you lift your hips up off the floor. On an inhalation, release your hips back down. Continue with this easy lifting and lowering for about five breaths; exhale your hips up as high as they comfortably can go, and then inhale and roll the spine back down, bringing the hips back to the earth. If you want more of a challenge, stay in the up position for a few slow, easy breaths. Be sure your head is on straight, with your chin in line with the little notch in the middle of your collarbones. And don't hold your breath!

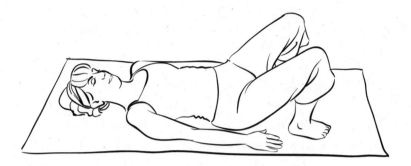

Figure 5.33a. Bridge Pose: Prep

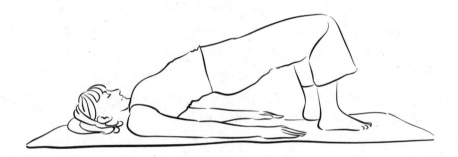

Figure 5.33b. Bridge Pose

When you're finished, stretch out your back by hugging your knees to your chest in both-knees-to-chest pose (posture 11). Remember, if it feels like a strain on your shoulders to hug your legs, please use a strap to catch your legs so you can keep your shoulders resting comfortably on the floor. Bring your awareness and your breath to your back, feeling the stretch in the muscles you've been working in the back of your body, letting your breath help these muscles lengthen and release. If you'd like, rock gently from side to side, giving your back a little massage.

deep relaxation

38. **Savasana:** The Sanskrit name for this posture means "corpse pose," and it looks pretty simple since, after all, you're lying still, doing nothing. But it's actually among the most difficult poses to master because it requires *totally* letting go of all physical tension, quieting the mind, and surrendering completely to the earth. So take a moment to set up this pose as carefully as you would a more-active posture. Consider setting a timer for five to ten minutes, or as long as you'd like to practice this relaxation pose, so you can completely let go and enjoy the experience without checking a clock to see if it's time to move on to other obligations.

Lie down on your back, with your legs straight and your arms resting at your sides about six to eight inches away from your body. If you feel any tension or tightness in your back, place a rolled blanket or bolster under your knees to help ease any discomfort. If you'd like, place a small folded towel or blanket under your head, making sure that, if you were viewed from the side, your forehead and chin would be about the same height so you can maintain the natural curve in your neck. You might enjoy placing a small eye pillow filled with flaxseed on your eyes. This can help deepen your relaxation by blocking out light and stilling involuntary eye movements. Consider covering yourself with a blanket since we often get cold when relaxing. Staying warm and comfortable will help you release tension and let go, which is the challenge of this deceptively difficult posture.

Let your legs be about hip-width apart and allow them to splay open comfortably. Roll your palms toward the sky if that's comfortable. If not, it's fine to let them face in or down. Be sure your head is on straight, with your chin in line with the little notch in the middle of your collarbones. Do any fidgeting you need to do and make any adjustments you need to make to become as comfortable as you can possibly be right now. Then come into stillness.

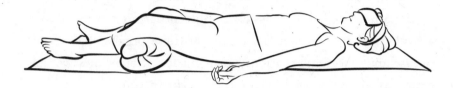

Figure 5.34. Savasana

When you're ready, please bring your awareness to your face and all the muscles of expression: the smiling and frowning, the excitement and the worry. As best you can, soften and relax all your facial muscles, allowing your face to be soft and passive.

Bring your awareness to your eyes, inviting them to rest softly in their sockets.

Bring your awareness to your brain, inviting it to rest softly in your skull.

With your mind's eye, release the hinge of your jaw so that your teeth gently part and your lips barely touch. Allow your tongue to fall from the roof of your mouth, and soften the inside of your mouth.

Bring your awareness to your head and let its weight drop completely into the earth, allowing your neck to relax, release, and let go. Soften and release your throat.

Bring your awareness to your shoulders; freed of the weight of the head and neck, your shoulders can rest back. If you feel any other burdens on your shoulders (many of us carry the weight of the world there), give yourself permission to set those burdens aside—just for now—and rest back.

Bring your attention to your arms, hands, and fingers; relaxing, releasing, and letting go.

Bring your attention to all your internal organs: the heart resting in the embrace of the lungs, the stomach, the kidneys, and all the other internal organs. Give yourself permission to let go of any physical tension you feel in any of these organs, and also to release any emotional tension you might feel. Sometimes we hold emotions in our organs; maybe there's fear in your belly, anger in your heart, or sadness in your lungs. Please give yourself permission to let go of *anything* that doesn't serve you at this time.

Bring your awareness to your hips, your buttocks, and your groin; relaxing, releasing, and letting go.

Bring your awareness to your thighs and knees; your shins and your calves; your ankles, feet, and toes—relaxing, releasing, and surrendering completely to the earth.

Bring your attention to your skin all over your body; allow it to relax, release, and let go.

Bring your attention to your muscles all over your body—relaxing, releasing, and letting go.

Allow your bones to become heavy and fall to the earth. Invite your flesh to soften away from your bones. Trust the floor to hold you up! Trust that everything is as it should be. There's nothing you need to do and nowhere you need to go. Rest here for as long as you'd like, thinking only of breathing out and breathing in. If your mind starts to chatter, please let those thoughts go, and come back to your breath. For now, there's nothing to do but relax, release, and surrender completely to the earth.

When your timer sounds and you're ready to come out of the pose, be sure to *slowly* bring your attention back to the room. When you're ready, bring gentle movement to your fingers and toes, and stretch any places that need to stretch. In your own time, bend one knee or both and roll onto your side, resting there for several breaths to ease your transition back from deep rest to everyday life. When you're ready to get up, bring your hands and arms in front of you, and use their strength to press yourself up to sitting position.

concluding your practice

Before moving on to your other obligations, take a moment for quiet reflection on the experience of your practice. You might want to offer thanks for the gift of breath and for anything else in your life that you're grateful for. Set an intention to stay connected to the sense of stillness and peace you've created with your practice. Recognize that this stillness is available to you at any time through your breath.

As you return to your busy day, see if you can carry this sense of stillness with you—and perhaps share it with others.

neck check:
eight essential
self-care strategies
for lasting relief

By now I hope you understand how yoga can empower you to relieve—and hopefully eliminate—pain in your neck and shoulders. And I hope it's also clear that yoga is not just a workout but also a comprehensive approach to self-healing and transformation that involves a variety of practices performed both on and off the yoga mat. While the practice of yoga postures is important to cultivate the strength, flexibility, and proper alignment essential to eliminating neck and shoulder pain, the simple practice of awareness throughout your day can also have a profound effect. Yoga asks us to pay attention to the many factors that can influence neck and shoulder pain—including our postural habits, body mechanics, thoughts, and emotions—and move with diligence and compassion in the direction of health.

And unlike other therapeutic options—such as going to a doctor, chiropractor, or acupuncturist—yoga is something that only *you* can do for *yourself.* While an experienced yoga instructor or yoga therapist can help guide you on this inner journey of self-discovery and self-healing, the practice is grounded in your own personal explorations and insights—and your connection with your own "inner teacher." Yoga is not a "one size fits all" endeavor. It's an individualized practice, tailored to fit your unique structure, background, personality, temperament, and needs. And it requires you to take responsibility for your self-care, an approach now recognized by Western medical experts as critically important for people with neck pain.

As a complement to the more detailed instructions presented in the rest of this book, I offer this concise summary of eight essential self-care strategies for healthy neck and shoulders:

on the mat

1. Regular Yoga Practice: Make a commitment to doing some formal yoga practice every day. By formal, I don't mean that you must necessarily put on a special outfit or spend a great deal of time. (See chapter 5 for specific recommendations on how long, where, and when to practice.) But it's essential to make your yoga practice a daily habit so that, even for a short time each day, you stop all the busyness of doing, planning, and striving so you can turn your attention inward, be present in your body, breathe, stretch, relax, and energize. While, ideally, this will take place on a yoga mat, circumstances may necessitate that your practice occur elsewhere, perhaps in a hotel room, in your office, or in bed. My teacher, Esther Myers, who died of cancer in January 2004, once told me that before she had cancer, she thought yoga postures performed in bed didn't count, that you had to do the postures on the floor for it to be yoga. But after her cancer diagnosis, she realized that it's all yoga.

on or off the mat

2. Breathing Practice: Slow, deep breathing is nature's own anti-stress medicine—and it's free, simple, and right under your nose. Breathing is the only bodily function that you can do either consciously or unconsciously and that's controlled by two different sets of nerves and muscles: voluntary and involuntary. When you take conscious control of your breath, it opens the doorway to relaxing your nervous system. Or, as yoga master B. K. S. Iyengar explains in his classic guide, *Light on Yoga*, "Regulate the breathing, and thereby control the mind" (Iyengar 1979, 21).

So take some time every day to focus on your breath. This can be part of your formal practice on the mat, or something you informally weave into your day, for example, while waiting at a traffic light or in a doctor's office, or anytime you feel stress. Some of my students tell me they use breathing practice to help them fall asleep at night or to get back to sleep if they wake up during the night.

Specific directions on deep abdominal breathing are offered in chapter 5. To deepen your experience, try these two basic breathing practices:

- *Even Breath:* Turn your attention to your breath, and mentally count the length of your inhalation and the length of your exhalation. Then try to make your inhalation and exhalation equal length. For example, you may count "one, two, three, four" on your inhalation and "one, two, three, four" on your exhalation. Or you may count to three, five, or six; it doesn't matter. Just do your best to make your inhalation and exhalation the same length. Continue for three to five minutes, and then let your breath return to its own natural rhythm.

- *Extended Exhalation:* Start with the even breath (above); then play with making your exhalation up to twice as long as your inhalation. For example, if you inhale to the count of four, try exhaling to the count of five, six, seven, or eight. As with all yoga practice, avoid strain. Just do your best to make your exhalation longer than your inhalation. This can be a particularly relaxing practice.

3. Meditation: If you've ever watched a beautiful sunset, stared at a candle flame, or gazed at a compelling picture or statue, you've practiced meditation. Despite the common misperception that meditation requires *emptying* the mind, meditation actually involves *filling* the mind with an object of focus, be it a flame, picture, flower, deity, color, sound, or virtually anything. Meditation is one of yoga's most important tools, as both a spiritual practice and a powerful healing methodology. Since the meditator seeks integration, becoming one with the object of focus, it's helpful to choose as your object of meditation something you find appealing that's also constructive, productive, and healing, such as an inspirational phrase or prayer. "The key is transforming the mind in a positive way," yoga master T. K. V. Desikachar told me when I interviewed him for an article in *Yoga Journal*, "because whatever happens in the mind happens in the whole system" (Krucoff 2007).

One of my favorite meditations is the following:

- *Mantra Meditation:* A mantra is simply a thought or intention expressed as a sound that's used as a focus of meditation. For your mantra, pick a word, a phrase, or a line of a poem or prayer that's meaningful to you. An example might be the Dorothy mantra: *There's no place like home.* Recite this mantra, either silently or out loud, once on your inhalation and once on your exhalation. Or, for a variation of the extended exhalation practice above, recite it once on inhalation and twice on exhalation. To begin, set a timer for three minutes and try to stay focused on your mantra the whole time. If other thoughts arise, notice without judgment that your mind is chattering and then return your focus to your mantra. Over time, you might try increasing the length of time you spend meditating.

off-the-mat practices

4. Integrate Yoga into Daily Life: Basically, this means *pay attention* to what's going on with yourself physically, energetically, mentally, and emotionally throughout your day.

Do your best to:

+ Sit, stand, and move with good posture.

+ Avoid staying in a fixed position for too long; get up and stretch, walk a bit, breathe.

+ Weave brief yoga "micro-practices" into your day. For example, do some simple postures at your desk (such as shoulder shrugs, hug arms, and seated back bend) or when you're standing in line (such as mountain pose, tree pose, and gentle twist). Get in the habit of taking a full, deep breath before you answer the telephone. Use waiting time—at a red light or while your computer boots up—as an opportunity to do a brief meditation.

+ Regularly bring your awareness to your neck and shoulders; perhaps set your alarm to ring every hour, and notice if you're holding tension in this area (including your mouth, face, arms, and upper back). If so, take a deep breath, and invite your muscles to relax and release.

5. Create a Supportive Environment: Be sure your physical surroundings support healthy posture—at work, in your car, and at home. Get the equipment you need to keep your neck and shoulders in good alignment, such as a telephone headset, and a properly fitted chair and computer desk with necessary accessories, like a document holder. Try to keep your energetic environment healthy by reducing clutter and mess. Cultivate a supportive social environment by strengthening positive relationships with people you care about and nourishing good friendships. If you find that your neck and shoulders become tense when you're around a certain person, avoid spending time with that person or work on improving the relationship.

6. Self-Study: One of the self-discipline practices (*niyamas*) outlined in the *Yoga Sutras of Patanjali* is *svadhyaya*, which means "study." This practice refers both to study of sacred texts and self-study, which is a vehicle for self-understanding and, ultimately, transformation. One of the best ways to learn more about yourself—your habits, thoughts, and emotions—is to keep a journal, a practice that's often recommended for people dealing with chronic pain. Consider keeping track of your pain level from day to day, perhaps using a 0 to 10 scale, where 0 is "no pain" and 10 is "the worst pain possible." In particular, note what you've been doing (physically, mentally, and emotionally) on days when you're experiencing high levels of neck and shoulder pain, and see if you can tease out the triggers connected to increased pain. In addition, you may want to write about stressful events and record your thoughts and feelings. The very act of reflecting on your life and writing down what you think and feel can be therapeutic. Writing in a journal may help you shed light on factors that contribute to your neck pain, learn about your own patterns of thought and behavior, and offer solutions for healing.

7. Self-Care Tool Kit: Certain tools can be useful in helping relieve pain, including:

- *Body tools:* Exercise balls, foam rollers, the Thera Cane, and other body tools can help you access particularly tight muscles and offer assistance in helping release tension. Consider using these tools in conjunction with breathing practice, inviting your muscles to release with each exhalation. (See the resources section for information on places to buy body tools.)

- *Ice packs:* I usually keep several soft ice packs in my freezer (available at most drugstores) for emergency first aid, since ice can be a safe and effective way to decrease inflammation and relieve pain. You can also use a bag of frozen peas or corn, which molds nicely around curved body parts like the neck and shoulders. Be sure to place a thin towel between your skin and the ice. People are often confused as to when to use ice and when to use heat for pain relief. The general rule of thumb is ice for a new or acute pain, and heat for an old or chronic pain. But even if it's a pain that's been around for a while, if you're having a flare-up, ice may be a good choice. Experiment and see which works best.

- *Heating pads and warm baths:* To soothe chronic aches and stiffness, consider applying heat by using a heating pad or soaking in a warm bath. To help relieve muscle aches, add Epsom salts and essential oils to the bath, using a relaxing fragrance such as jasmine or lavender.

8. Establish a Support Team: Build a network of health professionals who can help you meet your goals. Depending on your individual situation and needs, your network may include physicians, massage therapists, acupuncturists, physical therapists, chiropractors, psychotherapists, yoga therapists, and yoga teachers. But remember that you're in charge of your own health; view these professionals as your consultants and partners who offer you their wisdom and help you make the best choices for your own healing. Consider attending a regular yoga class, led by an experienced and well-qualified instructor (see the resources section for help finding one). Being part of a community of like-minded seekers, known as *sangha,* can be an extremely nourishing experience. But make sure that your yoga class is a complement to your regular home practice, not a substitute for it.

These self-care strategies are not "commandments"; they're not carved in stone! They're simply suggestions for steps you can take to harness the healing power of yoga. As always, use what works for you and ignore the rest.

And remember, be grateful that you *have* a neck and shoulders—even when they're painful. Be kind to them, pay attention to them, and do your best to take the necessary steps to cultivate healing in this challenging area—and in your entire body, mind, and spirit. Let each inhalation be an opportunity to fill your being with healing energy. And let each exhalation be a chance to relax, release, and let go of tension, pain, and anything else you don't need.

resources

---

recommended reading

Brantley, Jeffrey. 2007. *Calming Your Anxious Mind: How Mindfulness and Compassion Can Free You from Anxiety, Fear, and Panic.* 2nd ed. Oakland, CA: New Harbinger Publications.

Calais-Germain, Blandine. 1993. *Anatomy of Movement.* Seattle, WA: Eastland Press.

Coulter, H. David. 2001. *Anatomy of Hatha Yoga: A Manual for Students, Teachers, and Practitioners*. Honesdale, PA: Body and Breath Inc.

Desikachar, T. K. V. 1995. *The Heart of Yoga: Developing a Personal Practice*. Rochester, VT: Inner Traditions International.

Devi, Nischala Joy. 2000. *The Healing Path of Yoga: Time-Honored Wisdom and Scientifically Proven Methods That Alleviate Stress, Open Your Heart, and Enrich Your Life*. New York: Three Rivers Press.

Domar, Alice D. 2000. *Self-Nurture: Learning to Care for Yourself as Effectively as You Care for Everyone Else*. New York: Viking Penguin.

Faulds, Richard. 2006. *Kripalu Yoga: A Guide to Practice On and Off the Mat*. New York: Bantam Books.

Feuerstein, Georg. 2000. *The Shambhala Encyclopedia of Yoga*. Boston: Shambhala Publications.

Feuerstein, Georg, and Larry Payne. 1999. *Yoga for Dummies*. Foster City, CA: IDG Books Worldwide, Inc.

Finger, Alan. 2005. *Chakra Yoga: Balancing Energy for Physical, Spiritual, and Mental Well-Being*. Boston: Shambhala Publications.

Gaudet, Tracy W. 2004. *Consciously Female: How to Listen to Your Body and Your Soul for a Lifetime of Healthier Living*. New York: Bantam Books.

Kabat-Zinn, Jon. 1990. *Full Catastrophe Living: Using the Wisdom of Your Body and Mind to Face Stress, Pain, and Illness*. New York: Dell Publishing.

Kraftsow, Gary. 1999. *Yoga for Wellness: Healing with the Timeless Teachings of Viniyoga*. New York: Penguin Compass.

Krucoff, Carol, and Mitchell Krucoff. 2009. *Healing Moves: How to Cure, Relieve, and Prevent Chronic Ailments with Exercise*. Monterey, CA: Healthy Learning.

Lasater, Judith. 1995. *Relax and Renew: Restful Yoga for Stressful Times*. Berkeley, CA: Rodmell Press.

McCall, Timothy. 2007. *Yoga as Medicine: The Yogic Prescription for Health and Healing*. New York: Bantam Books.

Myers, Esther. 1997. *Yoga and You: Energizing and Relaxing Yoga for New and Experienced Students*. Boston: Shambhala Publications.

Payne, Larry, and Richard Usatine. 2002. *Yoga Rx: A Step-by-Step Program to Promote Health, Wellness, and Healing for Common Ailments*. New York: Broadway Books.

Scaravelli, Vanda. 1991. *Awakening the Spine: The Stress-Free New Yoga That Works with the Body to Restore Health, Vitality, and Energy*. 2nd ed. San Francisco: HarperOne.

Schatz, Mary Pullig. 1992. *Back Care Basics: A Doctor's Gentle Yoga Program for Back and Neck Pain Relief*. Berkeley, CA. Rodmell Press.

Stiles, Mukunda. 2005. *Structural Yoga Therapy: Adapting to the Individual*. San Francisco: Weiser Books.

audio and video

Kraftsow, Gary. 2008. *Viniyoga Therapy for the Upper Back, Neck, and Shoulders*. DVD (available at www.pranamaya.com).

Krucoff, Carol. 2008 *Healing Moves Yoga: A Mindful Practice for All Levels, with Carol Krucoff, RYT*. CD (available at www .healingmoves.com).

Payne, Larry. n.d. *Larry Payne's Yoga Therapy Rx: Common Upper Back and Neck Problems, Including Headaches*. DVD (available at www.samata.com).

Rothenberg, Robin. 2008. *The Essential Low Back Program: Relieve Pain & Restore Health*. Five CDs and book. Pacific Institute of Yoga Therapy (available at www.piyogatherapy.com).

yoga teachers and therapists

Yoga Alliance is an organization that registers both individual yoga teachers and yoga teacher training programs (schools) that have complied with minimum educational standards. For referrals to yoga instructors in your area, visit their website, www.yoga alliance.org.

International Association of Yoga Therapists supports research and education in yoga and serves as a professional organization for yoga teachers and yoga therapists worldwide. To find a yoga therapist in your area, visit their website at www.iayt.org.

Yoga for Seniors is codirected by Carol Krucoff and Kimberly Carson, and is a network of yoga teachers dedicated to making yoga practices available and appropriate for older adults. For more information, visit www.yoga4seniors.com.

yoga supplies and body tools

Hugger Mugger has provided yoga supplies for more than twenty years: www.huggermugger.com.

Bheka offers yoga supplies and healthy lifestyle products: www.bheka.com.

Barefoot Yoga Company offers yoga props, clothing, and accessories: www.barefootyoga.com.

Stretching Inc. Online offers a wide array of body tools, including the Thera Cane and the Knobble: www.stretching.com.

Orthopedic Physical Therapy Products sells a wide array of products used for therapeutic exercise, including foam rollers, gymnastic balls, and stretching straps: www.optp.com.

references

Benson, Herbert. 1996. *Timeless Healing: The Power and Biology of Belief.* New York: Fireside.

Brantley, Jeffrey. 2007. *Calming Your Anxious Mind: How Mindfulness and Compassion Can Free You from Anxiety, Fear, and Panic.* 2nd ed. Oakland, CA: New Harbinger Publications.

Butler, Robert. 2009. Phone interview by author, June. International Longevity Center, New York, www.ilcusa.org/pages/about-us/president-ceo.php.

Côté, Pierre, Gabrielle van der Velde, J. David Cassidy, Linda J. Carroll, Sheilah Hogg-Johnson, Lena W. Holm, Eugene J. Carragee, Scott Haldeman, Margareta Nordin, Eric L. Hurwitz, Jaime Guzman, and Paul M. Peloso. 2008. The burden and determinants of neck pain in workers: Results of the Bone and Joint Decade 2000–2010 Task Force on Neck Pain and Its Associated Disorders. Spine 33 (4S):S60–74.

Devi, Nischala Joy. 2000. *The Healing Path of Yoga: Time-Honored Wisdom and Scientifically Proven Methods That Alleviate Stress, Open Your Heart, and Enrich Your Life.* New York: Three Rivers Press.

Domar, Alice D. 2000. *Self-Nurture: Learning to Care for Yourself as Effectively as You Care for Everyone Else.* New York: Viking Penguin.

Haldeman, Scott. 2008. Phone interview by author, December. Department of Neurology, University of California, Irvine.

Haldeman, Scott, Linda J. Carroll, and J. David Cassidy. 2008. The empowerment of people with neck pain: Introduction— The Bone and Joint Decade 2000-2010 Task Force on Neck Pain and Its Associated Disorders. *Spine* 33 (4S):S8–13.

Haldeman, Scott, Linda Carroll, J. David Cassidy, Jon Schubert, and Åke Nygren. 2008. The Bone and Joint Decade 2000– 2010 Task Force on Neck Pain and Its Associated Disorders: Executive Summary. Spine 33 (4S):S5–7.

Hampton, Tracy. 2008. Improvements needed in management of temporomandibular joint disorders. *Journal of the American Medical Association* 299 (10):1119–21.

Hogg-Johnson, Sheilah, Gabrielle van der Velde, Linda J. Carroll, Lena W. Holm, J. David Cassidy, Jaime Guzman, Pierre Côté, Scott Haldeman, Carlo Ammendolia, Eugene Carragee, Eric Hurwitz, Margareta Nordin, and Paul Peloso, 2008. The burden and determinants of neck pain in the general population: Results of the Bone and Joint Decade 2000–2010 Task Force on Neck Pain and Its Associated Disorders. *Spine* 33 (4S):S39–51.

Hurwitz, Eric L., Eugene J. Carragee, Gabrielle van der Velde, Linda J. Carroll, Margareta Nordin, Jaime Guzman, Paul M. Peloso, Lena W. Holm, Pierre Côté, Sheilah Hogg-Johnson, J. David Cassidy, and Scott Haldeman. 2008. Treatment of neck pain: Noninvasive interventions—Results of the Bone and Joint Decade 2000–2010 Task Force on Neck Pain and Its Associated Disorders. *Spine* 33 (4S):S123–52.

Insurance Institute for Highway Safety. 2009. Q&As: Neck injury. www.iihs.org/research/qanda/neck_injury.html (accessed July 23, 2009).

Iyengar, Bellur Krishnamachar Sundararaja (B. K. S.) 1979. *Light on Yoga: Yoga Dipika*. Rev. ed. New York: Schocken Books.

Lasater, Judith Hanson. 2004. In Carol Krucoff, Anywhere, anytime yoga. *Prevention*, October, 113–18.

Lidgren, Lars. 2008. Preface: Neck pain and the decade of the bone and joint 2000–2010. *Spine* 33 (4S):S1–2.

McCall, Timothy. 2007. *Yoga as Medicine: The Yogic Prescription for Health and Healing*. New York: Bantam Books.

Krucoff, Carol. 2007. Positively healing: Everything that happens in your mind is reflected in your body, says T. K. V. Desikachar. *Yoga Journal*, 3 (201):111–15.

Mental Health Foundation. 2009. More fearful UK society linked to rise in anxiety disorders, says new report. www.mental health.org.uk/media/news-releases/news-releases-2009/14-april-2009/?locale=en (accessed July 22, 2009).

Myers, Esther. 1996. *Yoga and You: Energizing and Relaxing Yoga for New and Experienced Students.* Boston: Shambhala Publications.

National Center for Complementary and Alternative Medicine (NCCAM). 2008. Yoga for health: An introduction. http://nccam.nih.gov/health/yoga/introduction.htm (accessed July 6, 2009).

Sherman, Karen J., Daniel C. Cherkin, Janet Erro, Diana L. Miglioretti, and Richard A. Deyo. 2005. Comparing yoga, exercise, and a self-care book for chronic low-back pain: A randomized, controlled trial. *Annals of Internal Medicine* 143 (12):849–56.

U.S. Department of Health and Human Services (Physical Activity Guidelines Advisory Committee). 2008. Physical Activity Guidelines Advisory Committee Report, 2008. Washington, DC: U.S. Department of Health and Human Services. www .health.gov/paguidelines/Report/pdf/CommitteeReport.pdf (accessed January 8, 2010).

Carol Krucoff, E-RYT, is a yoga therapist at Duke Integrative Medicine in Durham, NC, and codirector of the Therapeutic Yoga for Seniors teacher training. An award-winning journalist and fitness expert, Krucoff served as founding editor of the health section of The *Washington Post*, where her syndicated column, *Bodyworks*, appeared for twelve years. A frequent contributor to *Yoga Journal*, she has written for numerous national publications, including The *New York Times*, *Prevention*, and *Reader's Digest*, and is creator of the home practice CD, *Healing Moves Yoga*. Krucoff is certified as a personal trainer by the American Council on Exercise. She also has earned a second-degree black belt in karate and sits on the peer review board for the International Journal of Yoga Therapy. She has practiced yoga for more than thirty years.

Foreword writer **Tracy W. Gaudet, MD,** is executive director of Duke Integrative Medicine and assistant professor of obstetrics and gynecology in the Duke University Health System. Author of the highly acclaimed *Consciously Female*, Gaudet is a practicing, board-certified OB/GYN and was the founding executive director of Dr. Andrew Weil's Program in Integrative Medicine at the University of Arizona. She lives with her son Ryan in Durham, NC.

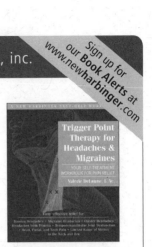
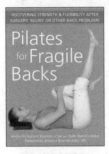
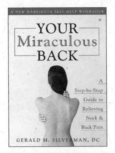
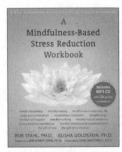
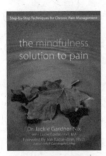
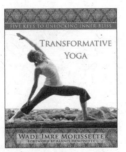

yoga to ease your aching neck & shoulders

Everyday activities such as using the computer, driving, or even curling up with a good book can create tension in the neck and shoulders. It's no wonder that so many of us have persistent discomfort and pain in these areas. *Healing Yoga for Neck and Shoulder Pain* presents simple, yoga-based practices that you can do at work and at home to release muscle tension for immediate relief.

After suffering from chronic neck pain for years, author and yoga therapist Carol Krucoff developed the unique self-care program found in this book. Now you, too, can free your ~~~~~~ eck pain by practicing simple yoga exercises to str~~~~~~~~~ ~~~~~~~ngthen weak ones and by learning to properly ali~~~~~~~~~ ~~~~ performing everyday activities that may be contributing ~~ your pain. This fully illustrated, easy-to-follow guide-book also addresses common problems that may accompany neck tension, including headaches, upper back pain, and stress.

> "I recommend it enthusiastically as a friendly vehicle anyone can use to explore and experience the amazing power and healing potential of these human bodies." —JEFFREY BRANTLEY, MD, director of the Mindfulness-Based Stress Reduction Program at Duke Integrative Medicine

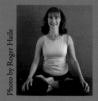

Photo by Roger Haile

CAROL KRUCOFF, E-RYT, is a yoga therapist at Duke Integrative Medicine in Durham, NC, where she creates individualized yoga practices for people with health challenges. She is also an award-winning journalist.

Foreword writer TRACY W. GAUDET, MD, is executive director of Duke Integrative Medicine and was the founding executive director of Dr. Andrew Weil's Program in Integrative Medicine at the University of Arizona.

ISBN 13: 978-1-57224-712-3

newharbingerpublications, inc.
www.newharbinger.com

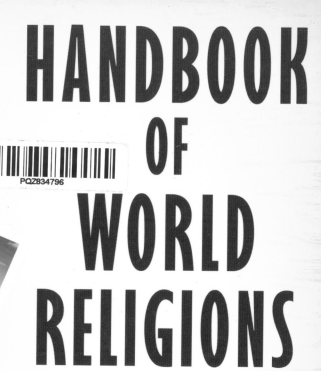

HANDBOOK OF WORLD RELIGIONS

Worldviews

...

Brief Histories

...

Basic Beliefs and Values

...

Major Differences with Christianity

...

Full-Color Illustrations

LEN WOODS

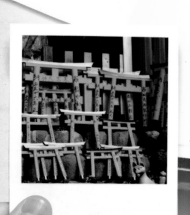